Praise for
Winter Blues

"I hibernated every winter, and sleeping in later and later caused all sorts of problems in my life. Dr. Rosenthal's advice helped me break the cycle and reset my biological clock. This book does a great job of breaking down complicated science into doable action items to improve my life during the dark winter days." —R. B.

"From the definitive expert on SAD, *Winter Blues* remains the go-to, authoritative resource. If you have suffered with symptoms for years, read this book—your life can be less of a seasonal roller coaster. In a warm, accessible style that is a pleasure to read, Dr. Rosenthal arms you with the information and tools you need to feel better across the seasons."
—KELLY J. ROHAN, PHD, author of *Coping with the Seasons*

"SAD sufferers worldwide owe Dr. Rosenthal a huge debt of gratitude, not only for pioneering SAD treatments, but also for writing and regularly updating this key book. The fourth edition is bang up to date, with many changes from previous editions, and remains fresh and interesting to read." —JENNIFER EASTWOOD, Honorary Life President, U.K. SAD Association

"This book has helped me to recognize my own seasonality, and its practical advice has offered me hope for a happier, more productive future. It was exciting to gain a better understanding of my own behavioral patterns. I've already begun to incorporate Dr. Rosenthal's recommendations into my daily regimen." —C. W.

"Dr. Rosenthal was among the tight team of clinical researchers who first discovered SAD in the 1980s, and he has led the field ever since. Readers of the fourth edition will find a treasure trove of fascinating scientific information combined with invaluable practical guidance for overcoming this common, much-misunderstood problem."
—CHRIS THOMPSON, MD, FRCP, FRCPSYCH, Chief Medical Officer, Priory Hospitals Group, United Kingdom

"A highly enjoyable book on SAD, written by the clinical scientist who has probably done the greatest amount of work on it."
—*Journal of Clinical Psychiatry*

Winter Blues

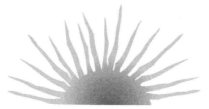

Winter Blues

FOURTH EDITION

Everything You Need to Know
to Beat Seasonal Affective Disorder

NORMAN E. ROSENTHAL, MD

THE GUILFORD PRESS
New York   London

Published by The Guilford Press
A Division of Guilford Publications, Inc.
72 Spring Street, New York, NY 10012
www.guilford.com

Library of Congress Cataloging-in-Publication Data

Rosenthal, Norman E.
   Winter blues : everything you need to know to beat seasonal affective disorder / Norman E. Rosenthal. — 4th ed.
      p.   cm.
   Includes bibliographical references and index.
   ISBN 978-1-60918-185-7 (pbk. : alk. paper) — ISBN 978-1-4625-0570-8 (hardcover : alk. paper)
   1. Seasonal affective disorder—Popular works.   2. Phototherapy—Popular works.   I. Title.
   RC545.R67 2013
   616.85'27—dc23
                                                                      2012014200

For Leora, Josh, and Liana

Contents

Part I
Seasonal Syndromes

Part II
Treatments

Part III
Celebrating the Seasons

Part IV
Resources

Preface

Welcome to the fourth edition of *Winter Blues*. Those of you familiar with earlier editions will find many updates in this book, particularly in the area of light therapy. Also, I have added a substantial chapter on meditation for seasonal affective disorder (SAD) and the milder winter blues, reflecting my belief in its ability to reduce stress, especially at a time when many of us are so vulnerable to the stresses and strains of everyday life. But I have also tightened the book up considerably, omitting elements including the history of the condition over the centuries, poetry about SAD, and nutritional advice on reducing high-impact carbohydrates from the diet. (Such advice is now readily available from many other sources.)

For those of you who have not read previous editions of *Winter Blues*, I hope you will find that the book lives up to its subtitle—*Everything You Need to Know to Beat Seasonal Affective Disorder.*

In deference to the fast-paced lives that most of us lead, the book is full of bullets, boxes, and tables to help you access the information you need as efficiently as possible. At the same time, I have preserved the conversational style that people have told me has worked for them over the years. I hope it works for you too and that you find the book helpful.

Winter Blues

Introduction

Whoever wishes to pursue the science of medicine in a
direct manner must first investigate the seasons of the
year and what occurs in them.

—HIPPOCRATES

Four seasons fill the measure of the year;
There are four seasons in the mind of man.

—JOHN KEATS

> ▸ **When the dark days of winter approach, do you feel slowed down? Do you have difficulty waking up in the morning?**
>
> ▸ **Are you tempted to snack more on those holiday foods, and do you find the pounds begin to creep on even as you valiantly try to diet?**
>
> ▸ **Do you find it hard to focus at work or in your relationships or feel down in the dumps or, worse still, really depressed?**

*I*f you answered yes to one or more of these questions, you may be one of the millions of people who have problems with the changing seasons. One of the astonishing facts to emerge from recent research is that most people in the northern United States and Europe experience seasonal changes in mood and behavior, also known as seasonality. In its most marked form, affecting an estimated 5% of the U.S. population, seasonality can actually cause a great deal of distress and difficulties in functioning both at work and in one's personal life. These estimated 14 million Americans are said to be suffering from seasonal affective disorder, or SAD, a condition now generally accepted by the medical community and the public at large. Another 14% of the adult U.S. population is estimated to suffer from a lesser form of SAD, known as the winter blues. Though these people are not usually affected severely enough to seek medical attention, they nevertheless feel less cheerful, energetic, creative, and productive during the dark winter days than at other times of the year.

For the last 30 years, I have studied the seasons and their effects on myself and others. I have loved them and hated them. I have helped others struggle with and master them, even as I have often struggled with them myself. This book is written for all of you who are intrigued by the changing seasons and their effects on our minds and bodies, whether this interest derives from medical necessity, a wish to understand or help a loved one, or plain and simple curiosity. Like the bears, squirrels, and birds, humans have evolved under the sun. We incorporated into the machinery of our bodies the rhythms of night and day, of darkness and light, of cold and warmth, of scarcity and plenty. Over hundreds of thousands of years, the architecture of our bodies has been shaped by the seasons and we have developed mechanisms to deal with the regular changes that they bring. Sometimes, however, these mechanisms break down and cause us trouble.

The effects of the seasons on humans have been well known through the centuries to artists, poets, and songwriters. Shakespeare, for example, observed that "a sad tale's best for winter," while Keats wrote of a nightingale singing of summer "in full-throated ease," and the singer of a well-known ballad calls his beloved the sunshine of his life. They have also been part of our ordinary language and culture. A person might be said to have a warm and sunny disposition or a dark and icy nature. The weather reports that are part of every television news program may be as much a way of helping viewers gear their mind-set accordingly as advising them on how to dress or whether to wear a raincoat.

In recent years, science and medical practice have caught up to some extent with language, culture, and the arts, and the medical importance of the seasons is starting to be appreciated. Signs of this are everywhere in evidence. For example, on January or February evenings, after the Christmas lights have been removed, a blue-white light can be seen streaming through the blinds and shutters of homes in neighborhoods throughout the North, penetrating the inky darkness of the winter night. The fanciful might mistake this strange illumination, brighter than the incandescence of an ordinary electric light and of a different hue, for an alien spaceship landed in suburbia to investigate our peculiar human ways or conquer our planet. The real explanation is more mundane. Thousands of people across the country are sitting in front of light boxes, specially made fixtures that emit far more light than is ordinarily available indoors, to treat their symptoms of SAD and its milder variants. Such boxes are springing up in offices as well, as many people, unashamed of their hibernating status, are treating their symptoms while at work.

But it is not only those who suffer badly as a result of the changing seasons who are becoming more cognizant of the importance of light. Having an office with a window has taken on a new importance as workers, who always wanted a view, now realize that there are medical and psychological benefits as well to having access to natural light. The "energy-efficient" buildings with tinted-glass windows constructed in earlier decades are now regarded with displeasure by many who must labor in the unnatural glow of the light transmitted through yellow panes. In fact, in one government building near Washington, the workers mutinied and pulled the tinted "weather stripping" off the outside of the windows to let in the sunlight unimpeded.

In Part II of this book, I will describe in detail how you can use light therapeutically as well as many other ways to treat SAD or the winter blues. I must emphasize, though, that depression can be a serious illness: painful, debilitating, and, in some cases, even fatal. If you think that you may be suffering from a seasonal form of depression and are taking steps to combat it yourself—which may be a critical first step—and this approach does not promptly take care of the problem, I recommend that you consult a professional sooner rather than later. There are so many things that can be done to alleviate depression, and a skillful practitioner can be an invaluable and sometimes essential ally in helping to implement these strategies. Your primary care physician or local university department of psychiatry may be a useful resource in directing you to a knowledgeable professional, should that prove necessary.

An enormous amount of research into the effects of the seasons and of light on human beings has appeared over the last few decades. Much of this research is based on the dramatic seasonal changes that occur in animals. I will describe some of these exciting new advances, which explain why some people experience seasonal changes so much more profoundly than others. I will also discuss the research conducted to explain how light therapy and other treatments may exert their dramatic therapeutic effects and also discuss the use of light therapy for other conditions. A chapter specifically written for this edition describes the potentially valuable role of meditation in helping to combat the winter blues.

But it would be a shame if the seasons were considered merely a source of suffering and distress. Aside from their capacity to induce symptoms, the seasons fascinate in their own right. The predictable changes that come with the shortening and lengthening of the days, the marked shifts in weather, and the rhythmic alternation between the barren landscape of winter and the vivid colors of summer are a continuing source of wonder.

The seasons of the mind are not the same for everyone. Autumn enchants some with its grand colors, but for others it carries the menace of winter. For certain people, winter, cheerless and forbidding, is associated with stagnation, decay, and loss. But others experience a different type of winter—one that finds them snug and cozy by the fireside, with chestnuts popping. Spring brings buds and blossoms, rebirth, with sap stirring, feverish urges, and a longing to go on pilgrimages. But we are also told that "April is the cruelest month ... mixing memory and desire." Summer yields a harvest of fruit and flowers, but according to Shakespeare, "sometimes too hot the eye of heaven shines."

In Part III, "Celebrating the Seasons," I discuss how the cycle of the seasons has shaped the way we think and inspired some of our most venerated works of art throughout history. In Chapter 16 I explore the connection between mood disorders like SAD and creativity.

In the final chapter, "Winter Light," I discuss life beyond SAD. By now, there are many of us who have suffered winter difficulties in the past but have successfully treated ourselves for years and have largely overcome the problem. I regard myself as lucky to be living after the recognition of SAD and the discovery of light therapy and other effective treatment strategies. Many people with SAD enjoyed the winters of their childhood before their symptoms first appeared. Then they suffered for years until they understood the nature of their problem and found successful treatments for it. After their SAD symptoms had been treated for several years, they began to rediscover the quiet pleasures of winter and to feel reconnected with their childhood. I relate some of their stories—and my own—and celebrate the joy of winter that has eluded so many of us for so long.

How to Use This Book

This book is intended to be a comprehensive volume covering every aspect of SAD that I believe readers might be interested in learning about. There are different paths you can take through the book, and some of you may not want or need to read it from cover to cover, in order. What you read now may depend on whether you are just starting to explore SAD or hoping to hone your current treatment. Your need for information or advice may change over time as well, and I hope you will come back to the book whenever you have new questions or new life circumstances that call for a modification of your approach to addressing your symptoms of SAD.

If you are just discovering (or beginning to suspect) that you suffer from seasonality, you will find what you need to understand the syndrome and how to treat it effectively in Parts I and II. You might want to go right to Chapter 2, where you will learn about the symptoms and also read the personal stories of people whose experiences may resemble your own. Chapter 3 will help you get an idea of the severity of your symptoms so you can begin to decide what to do about them, from self-help to professional interventions. Part II will then give you up-to-date information on the effectiveness of various different types of treatment. I recommend that you read all of Chapters 7–11 to get an idea of the range of options available, since many people find that coming at SAD from several angles provides the greatest relief.

If you have known for some time that you have SAD, you might be looking for information on another type of treatment to add to your regimen and can pick and choose from the chapters in Part II as needed. Chapter 12 will help you look at the inevitable cycle of the year as a whole and plan how to navigate each season with the least disruption.

The other chapters in Parts I and II cover more specific concerns: If you have children, you might be particularly interested in reading Chapters 4 and 5 to get a better idea of the causes of SAD and the chance that your offspring may end up with SAD symptoms too. You'll learn the signs to watch for and what we know about treating SAD in younger people. If you have seasonality that does not quite fit the profile of the winter blues, you will find Chapter 6 illuminating and may discover that you have a different version of seasonality.

When I began my exploration of SAD in the early 1980s, I quickly became fascinated by how we all navigate and respond to the changes of season that occur year in and year out. To me, SAD falls near one end of a continuum along which we are all governed by the seasons. You can learn a lot more about the age-old relationship between light and many aspects of living in the rest of this book. The chapters in Part III can help you accept seasonality as part of being human and find ways to appreciate and take advantage of what you know about yourself and the seasons of the year. You might also want to read about the discovery of SAD (Chapter 1), which I had the great privilege to be part of. I hope that I convey to you the excitement I feel about ongoing discoveries regarding seasonality and the hope that you can have a better and better relationship with the seasons in the years to come.

Part I

Seasonal Syndromes

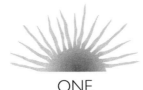

ONE

Discovering SAD

*W*hether by the diagnostic term "seasonal affective disorder" or the informal term "winter blues," you have probably heard about this condition.

SAD and Light Therapy: The Early Years

Although individual cases of SAD have appeared in the psychiatric literature for over a hundred years, and although the use of light to treat depression was suggested even in ancient times, the description of SAD as a syndrome and the systematic development of light therapy to treat it occurred as recently as the early 1980s, at the National Institute of Mental Health (NIMH). These developments involved several individuals, each of whom made an important contribution to the story. I consider myself fortunate to have been at that place at that time and to have played a key part in these events, which I describe below. And since each of us experiences our world from our own particular vantage point, it seems easiest to begin this tale of scientific discovery with my own SAD story.

My Own SAD Story

I trained as a doctor in South Africa, a country that, for all the turbulence of its politics, can truthfully boast about its climate. In Johannesburg, where I grew up, there were really only two seasons: summer and winter. During summer, one could swim outdoors and eat summer fruit: peaches, papaya, mangoes. During winter, one could not do these things. It was warm outdoors during the day, though at night you needed a sweater. Spring and autumn were transition times. After several months of winter, the blossoms would appear, and you knew it was spring. Likewise, when the long summer was over, the leaves would turn a simple brown and fall off the trees without much fuss or fanfare, and winter was there. But despite the mildness of the seasons, I was aware at some level of the effect they had on my mood. I had even considered writing a novel in which the mood of the central character changed regularly with the seasons. The novel was never written, but the seed of the idea stayed with me, germinating quietly. It required the intense seasonal changes of the higher latitudes to which I moved to activate that germ of an idea, as well as encounters with some inspiring people, who are central to this story. I arrived in the United States in the summer of 1976 and began both my psychiatric residency at the New York State Psychiatric Institute and research into disorders of mood regulation. The summer days felt endlessly long, and my energy was boundless. I had never experienced such long summer days in Johannesburg, which is far nearer to the equator than New York City.

As the months passed, I was struck by the drama of the changing seasons. I had been unprepared for the brilliant colors of the autumn leaves in the North, the crisp days and cold nights, and most of all, the disappearance of the light. I had not anticipated how short the days would be. When the sun shone, its rays struck the earth at a strange, oblique angle, and I understood what Shelley meant when he wrote:

> Bright Reason will mock thee
> Like the sun from a wintry sky.

Then daylight savings time was over and the clocks were put back an hour. I left work that first Monday after the time change and found the world in darkness. A cold wind blowing off the Hudson River filled me with foreboding. Winter came. My energy level declined, and I wondered how I could have undertaken so many tasks the previous summer. Had I been crazy? Now there seemed to be no alternative but to hang in and try to keep everything afloat. I understood for the first time the stoic temperaments of the northern nations. Finally, spring arrived. My energy level surged again, and I wondered why I had worried so over my workload.

I registered all these impressions, but I did not put them together into a cohesive story—and I probably would never have done so had it not been for the events that followed and the remarkable people I was to meet. At the end of my residency I went to the NIMH in Bethesda, Maryland, to undertake a research fellowship with Frederick Goodwin, whom I had heard speak on the topic of manic–depressive illness from both biological and psychological points of view. Goodwin made the subject come alive, describing how our shifting moods and fluctuating perceptions of the world correspond to certain changes in our brain chemistry. Since mind and brain seemed equally fascinating frames of reference, I wanted to use both models to try to understand mood disorders.

Shortly before my first visit to the NIMH, I met Alfred Lewy, one of several psychiatrists working with Goodwin at the time. Lewy had just developed a technique to measure the hormone melatonin, in collaboration with Sanford Markey. Melatonin is produced by the pineal gland, a pea-sized structure tucked underneath the brain. Each night, like clockwork, the pineal gland releases melatonin into the bloodstream in minute quantities and continues to do so until dawn. The secretion of melatonin signals the duration of darkness and thus serves as an important seasonal time cue in animals. Although it is unclear whether melatonin is instrumental in causing seasonal changes in humans, research in this area proved to be a critical step in the description of SAD and the development of light therapy.

Lewy and I spoke about our common interests and the various directions in which our research might take us. On occasion, we chatted over a mass spectrometer, the instrument he had used to develop his technique for measuring melatonin. It looked like a very large washing machine. He injected samples of clear fluid into a small hole in the top, and reams of paper rolled off it, while inked pens traced out a graph upon the paper. He pointed to one blip on the graph and said, "That's melatonin." I was suitably impressed.

After I joined Goodwin's group, I was assigned to work most closely with Thomas Wehr, an outstanding clinical researcher who had for some years been studying biological rhythms in an attempt to learn whether abnormalities in these rhythms might be the basis of the mood disturbances in depression and mania. Shortly before my arrival at the NIMH, Lewy and Wehr had shown that bright light was capable of suppressing the secretion of human melatonin at night—a finding that was to have great influence over the events that followed. There was a buzz in Goodwin's group at that time—a sense of excitement—and I felt certain I had come to the right place.

A Light-Sensitive Scientist

Although many people were responsible for the discovery of SAD, our steps toward this end can all be traced back to the actions of one man: Herb Kern. In some ways, Herb might have appeared to be an unlikely person to initiate a new area of medical investigation, for he was not himself a medical professional, but a research engineer with a major corporation. I met Herb a year after arriving at the NIMH. At 63, he was a youthful-looking man with a wiry build, a crew cut, and a twinkle in his eyes. He was intensely curious, and he had noted in himself a regular pattern of mood and behavior changes going back at least 15 years. A scientist by nature and training, he had kept careful notes of these changes in numerous small notebooks. He observed that each year, from July onward, his mood would decline and he would with-draw from the world. At these times, he lacked energy, had difficulty making decisions, lost interest in sex, and felt slowed down and "ready for hibernation." It was hard for him to get to work in the morning, and once there, he would sit at his desk, fearful that the telephone would ring, obliging him to have a conversation with someone. It is typical for a depressed person to withdraw—to have neither the desire nor energy to interact with others, which often seems like an impossible task. Depressed people simply want to be left alone.

More bothersome to Herb than his social isolation was his decreased creativity during his depressed periods. He would procrasti-nate at work because "everything seemed like a mountain" to him, and his productivity decreased markedly. It was only by grim perseverance that he was able to write up his research from the previous spring and summer. His sleep was disrupted, and his characteristic enthusiasm for life evaporated. The months would drag on like this for Herb until mid-January, when, over a two-week period, his energy would return. As he put it, "The wheels of my mind began to spin again." He had ample, even excessive, energy at these times and needed little sleep. Ideas came freely, and he was eager to communicate them. Over the next 5 or 6 months he would be very confident of his abilities, feeling as though he could "tackle anything." He was efficient and creative, needed only four hours of sleep per night, was more interested in food and sex, and acknowledged a "tendency to go overboard" in buying luxuries.

Herb had observed that his mood improved as the days lengthened and declined as they shortened, and he had actually developed a theory that this might be due to changes in environmental light. He attempted to interest several people in his hunch that his mood and energy levels were related to the time of year. One of these, Peter Mueller, a New Jersey psychiatrist in private practice who had a research background, listened to Herb and subsequently looked for other patients with a similar history. Herb was treated with several different antidepressant medications, all of which resulted in unacceptable side effects without correcting his symptoms. Herb read about the work of Goodwin, Wehr, and Lewy and found his way to the NIMH, where he asked us to work with him on his seasonal difficulties.

Lewy suggested that we treat Herb by lengthening his winter day with 6 hours of bright light—3 before dawn and 3 after dusk—in an attempt to simulate a summer day. He reasoned that since bright light is capable of suppressing melatonin in humans, it might also be capable of altering mood and behavior. This reasoning was strengthened by two observations: First, melatonin secretion is an important chemical signal for regulating diverse seasonal rhythms in animals; second, the nerve pathways involved in the suppression of melatonin secretion by light pass through parts of the brain that we believe are important in regulating many of the physical functions that are disturbed in depression, such as eating, sleeping, weight control, and sex drive. If the suppression of melatonin required light much brighter than ordinary indoor lighting, then perhaps bright light might also be necessary for the brain to perform certain mood-related functions.

We asked Herb to sit in front of a metal light box, about 2 feet by 4 feet. The box emitted as much light as one would receive while standing at a window on a spring day in the northeastern United States. We chose full-spectrum fluorescent lights—a type that mimics the color range of natural sunlight coming from a summer sky—to replicate the conditions that appeared to bring Herb out of his winter depressions. We covered the lamps in the light box with a plastic diffusing screen to create a smooth surface. Modern light boxes differ to some degree from the one we originally used in treating Herb. We now realize that it is unnecessary to use full-spectrum light and that, in fact, the ultraviolet rays present in some full-spectrum lights may actually be harmful to the eyes and the skin. In addition, newer light box models are smaller and more portable. Some models are tilted toward the person's eyes, an arrangement that produces less glare and is therefore more comfortable. Specific details about light boxes are provided in Chapter 7, "Light Therapy," and Part IV, "Resources."

Within 3 days, Herb began to feel better. The change was dramatic and unmistakable. He was moving into his spring mode several weeks ahead of schedule. Did we dare hope that we might have found a new type of treatment for depression? Intriguing as this possibility was, our excitement was immediately tempered by our scientific training. After all, Herb had been heavily invested in the light therapy. Might his response not have been a placebo effect? This effect has dogged behavioral researchers for years, and studies of light therapy would prove to be no exception.

A Human Bear

During the same winter that Herb was receiving light treatment at the NIMH, Peter Mueller, a private practitioner, in consultation with Al Lewy, tried artificial light treatment with another patient, whom we will call "Bridget." She also appeared to benefit from light and had an unusually good winter that year. The following summer, as luck would have it, Bridget moved to the Washington metropolitan area, and Mueller suggested that she contact us. Bridget's history and her ingenuity in translating the details of her seasonal problems into a coherent story were as remarkable as Herb's.

She was a professional in her mid-30s, who had been aware of disliking winter since childhood. But it was not until her early 20s that a regular pattern of seasonal changes emerged. Bridget's problem would begin each year in August or September, as she anticipated the forthcoming winter with increasing anxiety. What triggered this dread? she wondered. Could it be the fall catalogs, with their pictures of winter clothes? Regardless of the reason, when the leaves began to turn, she would feel a strong urge to take out her winter clothes and stock her cupboards with food, "like a squirrel getting ready for winter."

As winter approached, Bridget experienced many symptoms similar to those described by Herb, such as feelings of extreme fatigue—a leaden sensation that made her want to lie down and sleep all day. During these times, she had a marked craving for sweets and starches and overate. As with Herb, Bridget continued to struggle in to work each day, though her productivity declined markedly. When spring arrived, her depression lifted and was replaced by elation. In her earlier years, she would forget her winter difficulties once they were over. "I was like the grasshopper," she remarked, "singing and playing all summer long," indifferent to the next winter that was to come.

Bridget had also observed that other changes in the environment besides the seasons seemed to affect her mood. She had visited the Virgin Islands during the two winters before her first light treatment. Both times, her mood had improved markedly just days after arriving on the islands—only to relapse a few days after her return to the North. She had lived previously at different latitudes: Georgia, New York, and Quebec. The farther north she lived, the earlier her depressions began, the more depressed she felt, and the later were her spring remissions. She began to suspect that something in the environment was driving her mood changes—perhaps the light. Why else would she crave it so? Why else did she hate her poorly lit office? She made up any excuse to seek out the brightly lit photocopying room. Light treatment made good sense to Bridget. She was eager to try it and was delighted to find that it worked for her.

In Search of SAD

Unusual individual cases have historically played an important role in medical research in general and psychiatry in particular. We wondered whether Herb's and Bridget's symptoms might be examples of a special seasonal kind of depression and whether they might help us understand how others respond to the changing seasons and environmental light.

Although single cases may be of great importance in generating new hypotheses, we generally need groups of patients to test them experimentally. Mueller said he had encountered several other patients with seasonal depression. We wondered how common the problem was. Were there any other such individuals in the Washington, DC, area who might be interested in participating in a research program? I called a few local psychiatrists who specialized in treating depression, but they said they had not encountered the problem. I concluded that it must be quite rare and that the only chance we had of finding such a group was by publicizing our interest in the *Washington Post*. Sandy Rovner, a journalist who specialized in health issues, sat across the room from me, tape recorder in hand, and listened to my story. She decided it would be of interest to her readers and wrote an article for the *Post*, which launched an entire field of research. Rovner's article began with Bridget's own words: "I should have been a bear. Bears are allowed to hibernate; humans are not."

The response to the article took us all by surprise. Instead of our hearing from a handful of afflicted people, the phones rang for days and we received thousands of responses from all over the country. We sent out screening questionnaires, which were returned by the hundreds. I read them with a growing sense of excitement. In psychiatric research, heterogeneity is a major problem. In other words, the same condition may have diverse presentations and causes, which has proven to be an enormous obstacle to psychiatric researchers. As I read the questionnaires, it seemed as though Bridget had been cloned—one person after another reported the symptoms of the condition that we went on to call SAD. I wondered whether this uniformity in symptoms might reflect a common underlying biology, which might explain their favorable responses to light.

We interviewed many people and admitted into our program all those with clear-cut histories of winter depression. During that summer, as expected, all the participants felt well and showed an unusually high level of energy. This generated considerable skepticism among some of my colleagues, who speculated that we might be dealing with a group of suggestible people who had read the article and persuaded themselves that they had the syndrome. That seemed unlikely to me, but I had no way of disproving it, and could not help feeling slightly uneasy when one of my colleagues pointed out that if none of the participants became depressed when winter arrived, we would all look a little foolish.

The First Controlled Study of Light Therapy for SAD

The days grew shorter, and in October and November, right on schedule, the participants began to slow down and experience their winter syndromes, just as they had described. Although clearly not affected to the same degree as my seasonal patients, I noticed that I, too, had to push myself harder to get anything done. It was more difficult to get up in the morning, and even the project did not seem as exciting as it had the previous summer.

We planned to treat the patients with light as soon as they became moderately depressed—just enough so that we would be able to measure an effect of the treatment, but not so much that they felt incapacitated. We decided to use full-spectrum light, as we had with Herb Kern, for 3 hours before dawn and 3 hours after dusk. In any experiment designed to show the effectiveness of a treatment, it is important to have a control condition—one that incorporates all the ingredients of the "active treatment" condition except the element believed to be crucial for achieving the desired effect. In this study we believed that the brightness of the light would be crucial, so we used dim light as a control. To make the control treatment more plausible, we chose a golden-yellow light—a color associated with the sun.

We treated each patient with 2 weeks of one form of light and 2 weeks of the other form, then compared the effects—a so-called crossover design. More recent studies have used a so-called parallel design, in which different groups receive only one form of treatment. In all of these studies, it is important that those rating the response to treatment be "blind raters," meaning that they are unaware of the treatment condition for each subject. In the original SAD study, I was the only physician aware of the treatment condition, My collaborators, the blind raters, were Thomas Wehr, David Sack, and J. Christian Gillin.

I will never forget the first patient who underwent the bright light treatment—a middle-aged woman, markedly disabled by SAD. During the winter she was barely able to do her household chores, get to work, or attend her evening classes. After one week of treatment, she came into our clinic beaming. She was feeling wonderful, keeping up with all her obligations, and mentioned that her classmates were regarding her with a new competitive respect as she answered questions, as if to say "Where have you been hiding all this time?"

The second patient was treated with light around Christmas. I was on vacation and called my colleague Dave Sack to ask him how things were going with the study. "I don't know what treatment 'Joan' is receiving," he said, "but she's blooming like a rose."

And so it went. Nine patients responded to bright light, and the dim light proved ineffective. I began to use the lights myself and was sure that they made me feel better. Some of my colleagues requested them too. After a few weeks I had to put a big sign in front of the dwindling stack of light boxes, asking anyone who wanted to borrow a fixture to discuss it with me first so that we would have enough for the study. A local psychiatrist I had initially polled about the existence of people with SAD, who had told me that he did not know of any, called to say that he had realized that he himself had the syndrome and asked how he might use the lights himself.

Many questions were raised by the results of our first study. Was it really possible that light was affecting mood? Could there be some explanation for the improvement other than the light itself? Was it all a placebo effect? And if it was the light, how was it working? These were all important questions, and in due course, we and other research-ers would address them, one by one. But as we reviewed the study in the spring of 1982, we were delighted by its two main findings. The patients had become depressed on cue as they had predicted they would, and the light treatment had worked more dramatically than we had ever hoped it might. The azaleas and the dogwoods were in bloom. Spring had arrived, and at that moment, nothing else seemed to matter very much either to our patients or ourselves.

Thirty Years of SAD

Since our initial description of SAD and light therapy in the 1980s, we and other researchers have made tremendous strides in understanding and treating this fascinating condition. A recent survey of the literature showed well over a thousand publications on these topics. Throughout the world, scientists have found large groups of people suffering from the very same symptoms as our initial study subjects. We now know that SAD is common, affecting up to 9% of U.S. adults in the northern part of the country and in other northern regions such as Scotland. As one might imagine, it is far less common in the South, affecting, for instance, an estimated 1.5% of Floridians. To date, dozens of population studies have been undertaken to establish the frequency of SAD in different parts of the world.

In many instances the charge to educate people about SAD has been led by patients themselves. The highly successful patient support group SADA (Seasonal Affective Disorder Association) has been operating in the United Kingdom since the early days of SAD research. To date, unfortunately, efforts to organize similar SAD support groups have been less successful elsewhere. Despite the wealth of literature, market research indicates that clinicians still often fail to recognize SAD, thereby losing opportunities to alleviate the suffering associated with the condition. A large-scale study conducted by Jack Modell (then at GlaxoSmithKline), myself, and others, and published in 2005, indicated that people with SAD on average had suffered 14 winter depressions before entering the program. Of these, fewer than half had received any previous treatment for their symptoms. Why the lingering ignorance about SAD and its treatment decades after its initial description? Nobody knows for sure, but it may have something to do with light therapy itself, which continues to be viewed by many clinicians as outside the mainstream. This problem was highlighted by a 2005 lead article in the prestigious *American Journal of Psychiatry*. One encouraging development is that pharmaceutical companies have begun to take SAD seriously.

Three very large studies, encompassing collectively almost a thousand patients with SAD, indicate that the antidepressant Wellbutrin (bupropion) XL, if given before the onset of winter symptoms, can prevent an attack of SAD. These are exciting findings not only because they offer a novel approach to preventing symptoms, but also because they signify the entry of Big Pharma into this area. Historically, such corporate involvement has been important for the optimal recognition and treatment of other emotional conditions.

In 1987, the American Psychiatric Association recognized a version of SAD in its diagnostic manual, the DSM-III-R, and it can be found in the most recent version, the DSM-IV-TR. Now what we need is greater awareness among clinicians as well as the general public. My hope is that this book will continue to disseminate the valuable information that researchers have painstakingly garnered, fact by fact. The rest of this book outlines what we have learned so far about how the seasons affect us, what we can do to modify these influences, and some of the questions that have yet to be answered.

In Part I you will read about the following:

- The symptoms of SAD and how they may differ in type and severity in different people
- How to determine your own level of seasonal vulnerability
- How to pick up signs of SAD in children and adolescents
- Other forms of seasonal mood problems besides typical winter SAD.

I predict that future research will focus on continuing to find new approaches to treating SAD (the new chapter on meditation for SAD outlines one such attempt), as well as on new genetic studies of the condition. As with many other medical conditions, the discovery of genetic abnormalities may well point the way to novel treatments.

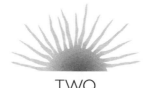

TWO

All about SAD

- ◗ What exactly is SAD?

- ◗ What are its symptoms?

- ◗ Who tends to get it and when?

- ◗ How long does it last?

- ◗ How does it affect the way people function at home, at work, and in their relationships?

- ◗ How does SAD relate to the "winter blues" that so many people complain about?

In this chapter I will introduce some key elements of seasonal disorders, as well as a few people who have suffered from them in their mild and severe forms—and triumphed over them.

We now know that, to a greater or lesser degree, the great majority of the population experiences some seasonal changes in well-being and behavior, in areas such as energy, sleep, eating patterns, and mood. At one end of the spectrum are those who have few, if any, seasonal changes. Then there are those who experience mild changes that can easily be accommodated in the course of their everyday lives. Yet another group finds these changes a nuisance—not worth taking to the physician, but troublesome nonetheless. This group may be suffering from what is commonly known as the winter blues. At the far end of the spectrum are people with SAD, whose changes in mood and behavior are so powerful that they produce significant problems in their lives.

Sketches of SAD

Such changes were well expressed by Jenny, who suffers from a typical case of SAD. She has observed that she feels like "two different people—a summer person and a winter person." Between spring and fall she is energetic, cheerful, and productive. She initiates conversations and social arrangements and is regarded as a valuable friend, coworker, and employee. She is able to manage everything that is expected of her with time and energy to spare. During the winter, however, her energy level and ability to concentrate are reduced, and she finds it difficult to cope with her everyday tasks. She generally just wants to rest and be left alone, "like a hibernating bear." This state persists until spring, when her energy, vitality, and zest for life return. It is easy to understand why she thinks of herself as two different people and why her friends wonder who the "real Jenny" is.

This theme is echoed by a variety of other seasonal people I have encountered. For example, a man from Missouri writes:

I feel as though I "live" only during the sunny months. The rest of the time I seem to shut down to an idle, waiting for spring, enduring life in general. This is no joking matter to those of us who are like this. We, in effect, live only half our lives, accomplishing only half of what we should. It is really rather sad, when you think of it.

One woman wrote about her elderly mother, who has suffered from SAD for her entire adult life:

In late spring or early summer, she is full of energy, requiring only 5 or 6 hours of sleep. She talks incessantly and tries to do too many things.

Then in late fall (occasionally she makes it to Christmas), her personality takes a complete turn. She sleeps 12 hours at night, cries all morning, and then takes a nap. She won't drive the car, seldom leaves the house, and won't answer the telephone.

Who are the victims of SAD? All sorts of people. The hundreds of patients with SAD I have known have come from all walks of life, races, and ethnic groups. One fact that has intrigued researchers for years is that the disorder is about four times more common among women than among men. Although people in their 20s through 40s appear to be most susceptible, SAD occurs in all age groups. I have encountered children and adolescents with the problem (see Chapter 5), as well as the elderly. In addition, SAD may affect different ethnic groups to a different degree (see Chapter 4).

Just as the degree of seasonal difficulties may vary from one person to the next, so may the timing of the problem. For example, one person may begin to feel SAD symptoms in September, whereas another will feel well until after Christmas. A more severely affected person might emerge from the winter slump only in April, whereas a mildly affected one may feel better by mid-March. Many people can predict almost to the week when they will begin to experience their winter difficulties and when they will begin to feel better in spring, almost as you can predict when different flowers will begin to bloom.

The timing of the appearance of symptoms also depends on where a person lives. My colleague Carla Hellekson, when she worked in Alaska, noticed that the patients in her SAD clinic became depressed about a month earlier, on average, than my patients in Maryland and began to feel better, on average, about a month later. Terry, a 38-year-old realtor, is typical of many who have lived at different latitudes when she reports that during her years in Canada and New York, her problems began earlier than when she moved south to Washington, DC.

Merrill, a vocational guidance counselor, sat in front of me, checking off on her fingers the symptoms she has during successive months. She had come to know her internal calendar well over the prior 18 years during which she had suffered from SAD. Since she was 32 years old when we spoke, these problems had been going on for more than half of her life.

I feel good for only 2 or 3 months: May, June, and July. By August my energy level has already begun to slip. I begin to sleep later in the morning, but I can still get to work on time. In September, things are a little worse. My appetite increases, and I begin to crave candy and junk food. By October I begin to withdraw from friends, and I tend to cancel engagements. November marks the onset of real difficulties for me.

I become sad and worry about small things that wouldn't bother me at all in the summer. My thinking is not as good as usual, and I begin to make stupid mistakes. Other people notice that I am not looking well. Preparing for Christmas is always an enormous chore. I am bad about getting my cards off and my gifts wrapped. I tend to avoid the usual round of parties: I don't want people to think I am being rude, but I find it very difficult to pretend to be cheerful and make conversation when all I feel like doing is going home and sleeping.

January and February are my worst months. On many days it's all I can do to get in to work, and often I don't. I call in sick. Once I'm there it's very hard to get my work done. I procrastinate as much as possible and hope that I'll be able to handle things later.

In March and April, my energy begins to come back, and that's a relief, but my thinking is still not back to normal, and I continue to feel depressed at times. They are tricky months, because you never know what the weather will be like. You can feel good for a few days and then, wham, you're down again. And then it's late spring and summer, and once again I feel myself: friendly and happy. I can do my work and can be available to the people I care for. But it's so hard to have to cram everything you want to do into 3 months.

In Washington, DC, the 3 months during which most patients with SAD feel like going into hibernation are December, January, and February. These months could well be called the SAD months. Then comes the thaw of March, April, and May. People emerge from their low winter state in different ways. Some glide gracefully through April and May into feeling cheerful and well in June and July. Some have a bumpy course over the spring, especially in places where it is dark, stormy, and unpredictable. Others emerge into an exuberant state where they may be excessively energetic, needing little sleep and feeling "wired" or "high." At times this state of excessive energy, known clinically as hypomania, can constitute a problem in its own right. A final group of people with SAD never quite emerge completely from their winter depressions and remain somewhat down all year round, though less so in the summer.

Elsewhere the pattern of SAD symptoms may differ. For example, in some more northern areas, symptoms may begin earlier, but may also end earlier if the ground is covered with bright snow, reflecting vast amounts of light on sunny winter days.

In Chapter 12, "A Step-by-Step Guide through the Revolving Year," I describe how many people with SAD feel during the different months and offer advice on how best to cope with the effects of the changing seasons.

Portraits of SAD

Following are profiles of four patients with SAD and one with sub-syndromal SAD. Their symptoms include the full range of seasonal changes. Neal and Angela suffered from milder and more common forms of SAD, which is why I profile them first, whereas Peggy, whom I profile second, suffered more severely. Finally, I profile Jeff, one of the first people with the winter blues to be studied and treated at the NIMH.

The people described in this section sought treatment shortly after SAD was first described, when light therapy was the major, if not exclusive, focus of therapy. They are of particular interest as they show just how powerful a treatment light therapy can be. Nowadays, even though light therapy is often a first-line treatment for SAD, it is standard to combine many different forms of treatment to achieve the best possible result. These may consist entirely of nondrug treatments (for example, light therapy, cognitive-behavioral therapy, and meditation) or could involve antidepressant medications as well. In Part II of the book, you will learn about other forms of treatment and read about people who have used different types of treatment in combination. An extreme example of this is "Sara: Throwing the Kitchen Sink at It" (pp. 227–228).

One myth I would like to dispel at this early stage is that SAD is always a mild condition—not a "major depression." Often I get asked, "What is the difference between SAD and major depression?" That's like asking, "What's the difference between cornflakes and breakfast cereal?" Just as cornflakes are a type of breakfast cereal, so SAD is a form of major depression. In fact, a 2003 Scandinavian study found people with SAD reported more symptoms of depression than those with nonseasonal depression who had recently been hospitalized following a suicide attempt.

The portraits that follow show people who have suffered from winter difficulties to differing degrees: Peggy most severely, Angela least severely, with Neal somewhere in between.

Neal and Angela: Light for a Living and Light to Write By

Neal Owens is currently the president of the SunBox Company, which sells lights for the treatment of SAD. He is in his mid-50s and has had difficulties during the winter for many years. His problems occurred in both his personal and professional life and affected the way he felt about himself.

Twice divorced, he feels now that his first marriage crumbled in part as a result of his seasonal changes. During the winter he was little fun to be around. He moped and withdrew into himself, was unable to enjoy the holidays, and was not available to his wife when she needed him. Then, single once again, he felt very bad about himself, and this was not helped by the 15 to 20 pounds he would gain each fall and winter. He would find it impossible to exercise at this time, losing yet one more source of enjoyment and means of reducing his weight and feeling good about himself.

In his work as a sales representative, he found his productivity declined markedly in the winter months. He would sleep late, cancel appointments, and spend much of the day at home, depressed. When he was able to get to work, he came home exhausted and would collapse on the couch for the rest of the evening. It is not surprising that for a salesman, who needs to be upbeat, energetic, and eager to interact with others and promote his product, the symptoms of SAD would be rather disabling.

He consulted a psychiatrist at the urging of his girlfriend and was given a series of antidepressants, none of which proved helpful. After seeing a television documentary about SAD, he mentioned light therapy to his doctor, who was not supportive of the idea. He then obtained information from the NIMH, constructed his own light box, and began therapy on his own. He switched therapists and improved noticeably, using a combination of light and psychotherapy. Neal's positive experience with light therapy inspired him to change careers and start a business to help others by selling light boxes and providing information on SAD. Neal now feels well all year round and is very hopeful about the future since his winter depressions are under control.

Angela is a 60-year-old writer with a long history of winter difficulties too mild either to meet criteria for a diagnosis of SAD or to lead her to seek medical help. Since her childhood, she has disliked winter and dark climates and places, which she has avoided whenever possible. She thought of herself as entering a "little hibernation" in the winter, when she would feel less creative than usual and "slightly melancholy," if not actually depressed. She had never consciously associated her low energy states with the quality of winter light, but when she first heard about SAD, she immediately identified herself as having a minor version of the condition.

Angela first found out about light therapy when she was writing a magazine article on the subject, for which she interviewed me. But she did nothing about her own winter problems until 4 years later, when she had strenuous writing deadlines to meet. She installed a set of lights on her desk, and they have been there ever since. She uses the lights in both summer and winter, whenever she happens to be working—at least when she is living in Washington, DC. She observes:

> Since I started using the lights in winter, my brain seems to be clearer, I seem to be happier, and the writing goes better. Not only am I much more productive, but I also seem to be much more creative. The words come more easily and I seem to get more images. I also don't mind being at my desk and writing as much as I did before. When I used to think of having to write in the winter, it was a great effort. I felt almost as though I would have to pull the resistant words out of my head by force and sheer will. Now I have a much lighter feeling about it. It's more fun.

In the last several years Angela has been so successful in her writing that she has purchased a second home in a popular Florida resort, where she spends much of her time—and she's happier and more creative than ever.

Peggy: Forty-One Grim Winters

Peggy is an attractive, youthful-looking woman in her late 50s with blue eyes, fair skin, and silver-gray hair. Retired now, she worked as a medical statistician for many years. She was married twice and now lives alone. She grew up in the Midwest and has had difficulty with the winter since she was 11 years old. She was always an excellent student. She would start out particularly well in the fall semester, but when winter came, there were always problems. Her teachers, who regarded her as one of their best students, would register surprise and dismay at the sudden change in her work. Her parents would also become "disgusted" with her performance, which would decline for no apparent reason.

This seasonal problem in school performance increased over time. In her senior year of high school she was an honors student and was given the responsibility for keeping a log of student aid contributions. The task involved simply putting a check mark next to the name of every student who had donated a nickel. Although she applied herself to the job enthusiastically in the fall, by the time November came, she found it overwhelming. Having such difficulties with so simple a task was confusing for Peggy but typical of her state of mind every winter. She scored above the 99th percentile on intelligence tests, but when she had difficulties with simple things, she believed she was a fraud and that the test results must have been wrong, that teachers must have given her good grades just because she was a nice person.

Peggy is sure that her mother had SAD as well. During the winter, her mother would nap most of the day, whereas in summer she was energetic and vivacious. Both Peggy and her sister were conceived in August. Winter seemed like a low time for the whole family, and Peggy's own difficulties went unnoticed by the other family members. These troubles reached a crisis during her junior year of high school:

> It was mid-January. There had been a string of gray days, but nothing bad had happened. I hadn't failed any exam or lost a boyfriend, but I felt so weighed down and in such a state of despair that I saw no future for myself. Everything I looked at was wrong. I went down into the basement, found a water pipe, got a piece of clothesline, and tried to make a noose out of it, but I was unable to do so. I just didn't have the energy to figure out how to do it properly or the strength to do it.

I went back upstairs to the bedroom I shared with my sister and lay down on my bed crying, disgusted that I couldn't even commit suicide properly. I kept the whole thing to myself. The next day was sunny and I said to myself, "Had you committed suicide yesterday, you wouldn't be alive to see this beautiful day," and I felt better. I always thought that it was a miracle that the sun was shining the next day. I wonder what would have happened had it been cloudy. That experience taught me not to try to predict the future—that one day can be bad and the next day good.

Although Peggy had thoughts of killing herself on several subsequent occasions, that was the only time she ever came close to trying.

During adulthood, Peggy's seasonal cycles continued. She would begin to prepare for winter in September, buying a 6-month supply of toilet paper and all other nonperishable goods, "like a squirrel about to hibernate." In November, she notes:

The physical difficulties start first: eating more, sleeping more, and the slowing down of brain functioning. Initially, I'm not sad. I can still sit down and laugh with friends and enjoy my favorite TV shows. As it becomes obvious that I'm less able to function at work or with friends, mental depression starts taking over. I have trouble writing Christmas cards, which adds to my depression, since I am unable to communicate with people I really care about. Even though I really don't want to lose touch with them, I simply want to be left alone from December until April.

Needless to say, this wish to withdraw caused Peggy difficulties both at work and in her personal relationships:

I worked in an office where there was a lot of gift giving. I would feel very upset with people who got their gifts out before December 20. I would wonder, "Why can't I get my gifts out on time?" By then I was closing the door to my office. I didn't want anyone to come in, and I would select only those phone calls I wanted to take. It was okay if people just wanted to chat, but I would hate it when they wanted me to dig up data or, worse still, to do a computer run. In the summer, doing that stuff was like a game. It was fun to sit in front of the computer. But in the winter any task was daunting.

The winter changes also caused problems in Peggy's relationships with men, in part due to her irritability and fault finding—common early signs of her winter depressions. She would drive to work in the winter "cussing out the other drivers." It was hard for her to believe that this was the same morning commute that she found enjoyable during the spring. The same relationships to which she was open in the summer seemed unappealing in the winter:

> I had several relationships with men I met in the fall, during the beautiful, sunny October days, and managed, because of the early passion of the relationship, to make it through the first winter. Summer was great. Then the next winter came along, and the relationship would collapse. In winter, when someone canceled an evening social engagement, I generally felt relieved and spared the guilt of having canceled the engagement myself.

The memory and thought-processing problems that troubled Peggy during her school and college days continued to cause difficulties later on. She would forget to set her burglar alarm, or where she had put the keys, or have problems with other things that she would take for granted in the summer. Every chore seemed to take much longer in the winter, and complex tasks, which were easy for her in the spring and summer, were quite impossible during the winter months. She would become anxious about her failures, irritated by her ineptitude, and accuse herself once again of being a fraud.

She would eat more in the winter, particularly carbohydrates. When she lived in the Northeast, she would have to drive home from work for an hour each evening through the gray New England landscape, and when she finally reached home, as she confessed to the minister at her church one Lent, she could not resist gorging on cookies. Was she not guilty of gluttony?

Her energy level stayed low all winter long. Over the years she developed strategies for coping. For example, she would buy lots of winter clothes and let the laundry pile up for months until the spring, when she could finally face doing it all.

Peggy's sex drive was low during the winter. She recalls with amusement how there were two workmen in the house one winter. In the late afternoon she was unable to stay awake, so she retired to bed and asked them to tell her husband that he could find her there when he got home from work. When he returned, he was incensed, "as though I were this terrible seductress who had gone to bed, tempting the workmen in the house. He felt as though I had destroyed his honor. I laugh when I think of it now. All I wanted to do was sleep, and the last thing I was interested in was seducing those men."

Peggy was in classical psychoanalysis for 3 years, "five days a week, every month of the year except for August," but the seasonal pattern of her problems never emerged as an issue for discussion in the analysis. She had no other formal treatment for her seasonal difficulties.

During the summer, she would often feel even more energetic and enthusiastic than the average person. Her high energy level would keep her working in the garden till 9 at night, and she would stay awake until 2 in the morning. She required only 6 hours of sleep. She recalls with amusement the summer day when she went rowing on a lake with a very large man. She felt so energetic that she did all the rowing, and the sight of a small woman rowing a 200-pound man across a lake caused a group of passing fishermen to whistle catcalls at him.

It was her winter depressions, not her summer highs, that brought Peggy to the NIMH Seasonal Studies Program. She was beginning to enter her November decline when she received a tax audit notice. The thought of having to collect and submit all the necessary records threw her into an intense depression and induced her to seek psychiatric help. She was 52 at the time and had suffered regular winter depressions for 41 years, though she had never recognized them as such. On being asked how that could have happened, she replied, "I thought it was normal to feel like that in the winter."

Peggy was treated successfully with light therapy. Shortly after treatment was started in January, she managed to refinance her house within a week—something she would never have been able to do before during the winter. After finding out about her seasonal problem, Peggy learned to take winter vacations in the sun. She moved into a house with large windows and decorated it in light colors. She entered weekly psychotherapy to deal with a variety of psychological issues. Having retired from her former job, she undertook a new career, working with elderly people. As a result of her treatment, Peggy now feels fulfilled and much happier with her life than ever before. When she thinks of what her understanding of SAD and her light treatment have given her, Peggy concludes:

Now I don't have to blame myself for what happened in past winters. It's liberating to know that SAD is a physical disorder—not my fault. I can give myself some leeway for what happens now. I don't have to be so critical of myself. I have a tool to make myself feel better.

Considering these three profiles of people with winter difficulties, I would diagnose Peggy as suffering from severe SAD, Neal as suffering from mild SAD, and Angela as having a case of the winter blues.

Together with Siegfried Kasper, who is currently Chief of Psychiatry at the University of Vienna in Austria, I set out to define this condition, which we formally called "subsyndromal SAD." We selected a group of people who, like Angela, were less productive and exuberant in the winter, but were never impaired to the extent that they would consider seeking medical attention. We found that far more people (an estimated three times as many) suffer from this milder version of winter difficulties than from the more severe version. Nevertheless, they still benefit from light therapy, just as Angela did.

We hypothesize that the winter blues and SAD are two broad categories of problematic seasonal change (also known as seasonality) to which many people are susceptible. Although some clearly fall into one category or another on the basis of the severity of their winter problems, many fall into a gray zone between the two. Bright light or other forms of treatment can help people in either category. The important distinction between the two is that those who are depressed should seek professional help, whereas those who are more mildly affected might reasonably consider trying to treat the problem themselves. Guidelines are provided in Chapter 3 to help readers decide when self-help alone might be reasonable and when to consult a physician.

It is important to realize how widely variable the severity of seasonal changes can be not only from one person to the next but even within the same person from winter to winter. One reason it is difficult to pin down the numbers of people with SAD and the subsyndromal winter blues is that a person could have full-blown SAD one year, winter blues the next, and be totally fine in the third year. In fact, I hope readers of this book who have suffered from winter difficulties will experience this type of progression after reading about the many available remedies for winter difficulties. For example, I no longer suffer from either SAD or the winter blues, no doubt as a result of heeding my own advice.

Diagnosing SAD

When clinicians or researchers diagnose a psychiatric condition, they use a set of standardized criteria. When we first described SAD, we needed to develop such a set of criteria. More recently, the American Psychiatric Association has established a different set of criteria, which are laid out in DSM-IV-TR (see Table 1). While these criteria are useful guidelines for clinicians and researchers, I would encourage you not to take them too seriously. If you experience some of the seasonal changes described in this chapter and find them problematic, you may well have SAD or subsyndromal SAD and may benefit from the treatments described in Part II of this book.

Core Symptoms of SAD

Although the individuals profiled earlier had very different experiences with seasonal difficulties, each had some manifestation of the core symptoms of SAD, described below in a little more depth.

CORE SYMPTOMS OF SAD

- Reduced energy

- Increased eating, including carbohydrate cravings

- Disturbed sleep

- Lowered sex drive

- Thinking problems, such as difficulty concentrating and processing information

- Mood problems, particularly depression

TABLE 1. Criteria for SAD

SAD criteria of Rosenthal et al. (1984)	DSM-IV-TR criteria for major depression with "seasonal pattern"
There is a pattern of winter depressions, at least two of which developed during consecutive winters.	There has been a regular temporal relationship between the onset of major depressive episodes and a particular time of the year.
At least one of these depressions was severe enough to meet the criteria for major depression.	In the last 2 years, two major depressive episodes have occurred that demonstrate the temporal seasonal relationship, and no nonseasonal major depressive episodes have occurred during the same period.
There are nondepressed periods in spring and summer.	Full remissions (or a change from depression to mania or hypomania) also occur at a characteristic time of the year (e.g., depression disappears in the spring).
No other major psychiatric disorder is present.	
There are no clear-cut recurring social or psychological reasons to account for the recurrent winter depression.	There is no obvious effect of seasonal-related psychosocial stressors (e.g., regularly being unemployed every winter).

Note. DSM-IV-TR criteria reprinted with permission from the *Diagnostic and Statistical Manual of Mental Disorders* (4th edition, text revision). Copyright 2000 by the American Psychiatric Association.

SAD as an Energy Crisis

Susan's description provides us with an important clue to an understanding of SAD and of depression in general. Many of the symptoms of depression involve physical functions: sleeping, eating, activity levels, sex drive. Disturbances in these functions produce physical symptoms, and their presence is an important clue that someone is suffering from a clinical depression and not just ordinary sadness. Often, in fact, the sadness and gloom that we associate with depression are not the most prominent part of the general picture. So important are the physical symptoms that modern diagnostic systems do not permit the diagnosis of depression if there has not been a history of at least some physical symptoms.

Almost all people with SAD have problems with their energy level, and they often express it in similar ways. Here are a few of their voices:

> *I don't really feel depressed. I just feel like all my systems have been turned off for the winter. I feel leaden and heavy and just want to lie about all the time. It's only when I am expected to do something out of the ordinary, and I realize I cannot do it, that I feel my mood being pulled down.*
> —Susan, a middle-aged homemaker, housewife

The fatigue is agony. I feel I have to drag myself from one place to the next.

Everything seems like more of a chore in the wintertime.

I have to use all my willpower just to get up in the morning, go to work, be pleasant to people, pay my bills, and put my dishes in the dishwasher.

Changes in Eating, Sleeping, and Sex Drive

Most people with SAD eat more in the winter and report a change in their food preference from salads, fruits, and other light summer fare to high-carbohydrate meals: breads, pasta, potatoes, sugary foods. Many have told me that eating carbohydrates actually makes them feel better, more energetic. Laura, a musician in her 40s, describes her seasonal change in eating patterns:

> *By September and October, I feel like I am constantly feeding and gnawing. My winter diet consists mainly of pastas, macaroni and cheese, rice casseroles, and chicken and mushroom soup—heavy, heavy food. Things that take a long time to cook so you smell them. Stews and pot roast with potatoes and gravy . . . lots of gravy on everything. And dessert—heavy dessert.*

Two research groups have actually tried to record the eating habits of people with SAD at different times of year. Judith Wurtman at MIT and Anna Wirz-Justice in Basel, Switzerland, have confirmed that the increase in carbohydrate consumption reported by so many patients does, in fact, occur. This pattern seems to be an exaggeration of the eating patterns in the population as a whole. One study performed in the cafeteria of the National Institutes of Health (NIH) found that people eat more carbohydrates in winter and more salads in summer. The same patterns were also found in a study conducted in Montgomery County, Maryland.

Bonnie Spring, now professor of psychology at University of Illinois at Chicago, showed that carbohydrates make nondepressed people feel more drowsy. But in an NIMH study, my colleagues and I gave high-carbohydrate meals (six big cookies)

People with SAD report that eating carbohydrates seems to give them more energy —the opposite of people who do not have SAD.

and high-protein meals (a plate of turkey salad) to people with SAD and nonseasonal people and found that the high-carbohydrate meal made the SAD group feel more energetic but the nonseasonal group more fatigued. This suggests that there is a basic difference in the brain chemistry of seasonal and nonseasonal individuals, resulting in a difference in response to carbohydrates.

We don't know for sure what this biochemical difference is, but studies of serotonin, a neurochemical messenger of widespread importance in brain functioning, may provide some answers. In a classic study, John Fernstrom and Richard Wurtman of MIT showed that in animals, dietary carbohydrates increase the production of serotonin in the brain. Further studies show that this mechanism may also occur in humans. One reason those with SAD crave carbohydrates and consume them in excessive quantities may be that they are responding to an instinct to correct a deficiency in brain serotonin transmission.

Another reason people crave carbohydrates may be that they secrete too much insulin, a hormone released from the pancreas. Insulin drives down blood sugar levels, which, in turn, may result in cravings for sweets and starches.

There is evidence from researchers in Basel, Switzerland, that people with SAD do indeed secrete too much insulin in response to dietary carbohydrates. When their depressions improve, during summer or after light therapy, this tendency to oversecrete insulin appears to subside. It is known that a tendency to oversecrete insulin can be quite unhealthy over time. It may signal a greater risk of diabetes, obesity, and heart disease in later life. It is therefore possible that treating SAD properly can be beneficial not only psychologically but also physically. In fact, there is an accumulating literature suggesting a connection between depression and cardiac disease.

Considering the changes in diet and the low levels of activity that occur in the winter in SAD, it is not surprising that people tend to gain weight, often quite dramatically. One physician with SAD tells me that his winter trousers are two sizes larger than his summer ones, and that is not unusual. I have seen people gain up to 40 pounds in the winter and lose it all the following summer. Unfortunately, some people do not lose it all and become steadily heavier from year to year. This yo-yo pattern of weight gain and weight loss has in itself been associated with serious medical conditions, such as diabetes and heart disease. Besides the strategies for treating SAD that I outline later in the book, I provide specific dietary advice to help readers avoid the carbohydrate binges and weight gain to which SAD sufferers are so often vulnerable.

People with SAD complain as much about changes in their sleep patterns as they do about their eating. Common problems are difficulty getting up in the morning, being tardy at work, and not getting the children off to school on time. People with SAD generally sleep more but don't feel refreshed on waking. Sleep is often interrupted and "low quality." Laura, the musician mentioned earlier, recalls seasonal changes in sleep patterns from her school days:

> I can remember being unable to get up in the morning during the winter as I was growing up, during high school, junior high. My mother would scream at me to get up and get ready for school. I would drag myself up. In contrast, during the spring, I would go out in the yard every morning before school started and look for a flower to wear in my hair or in my buttonhole. Obviously, I had to get up early enough to go and get the flower and have the desire to do that. In winter, I'd have a terrible time staying awake. . . . I used to work in the cafeteria, and I would get these baking powder biscuits at dinner. You could take home whatever was left over after dinner. So I would take a pile of these biscuits and a Coke. If you put a bite of biscuit and a sip of Coke in your mouth, it reacts and fizzes—that was how I stayed awake to study in the evening after I

would get back. I gained a lot of weight, but in the summer, the weight would come off—without dieting.

Flora, an editor in her mid-40s, describes somewhat different sleep patterns:

I'm tired all the time during my depressions, but I do have a little trouble going to sleep, so I'll read in bed for a long time. I never knew how often I woke up in the middle of the night until I started keeping track of it, but untreated, that's what I do. Then I would find it impossible to get up in the morning and would sleep through the alarm clock. Once, in college, I slept through a fire drill, which made my dorm mates very angry. The bell was right outside my room, and they all went out in the cold and stood there. But since I didn't go out, they had to repeat the fire drill. . . . This was in the winter.

Studies performed at the NIMH actually showed differences between the way people with SAD and nonseasonals sleep at different times of the year. In the winter, people with SAD sleep longer, as measured by electrical recordings of their brain-wave activity. They also have a decrease in a type of deep sleep called slow-wave sleep. The lack of slow-wave sleep, together with the greater number of sleep interruptions, may account for the daytime fatigue experienced by people with SAD during the winter, despite their increase in nighttime sleep duration.

In most people with SAD, sex drive decreases markedly during the winter. Many people report not wanting to be touched or to exert themselves in any way, but rather wanting to curl up and be left alone. I have heard many reports of women who wear long flannel nighties to bed during winter. While these garments are worn mainly for warmth and comfort, they may also communicate a lack of interest in physical intimacy on the part of the person with SAD. Likewise, men with SAD may lose sexual interest during the winter. Of course, shifts in sexual interest may also affect one's partner, who may easily feel rejected. When spring and summer arrive and the SAD sufferer's sexual interest picks up again, the couple will have to find a new equilibrium, which may be difficult. The person with SAD, forgetting that he or she has been uninterested in sex for several months, may be surprised at the partner's aloofness. The partner, who felt rejected or frustrated during the winter months, may eye the renewed sexual interest with suspicion or anger. An understanding that marked shifts in sexual interest are a common feature of SAD—together with communication between the partners about this problem—can greatly ease such tensions.

Sylvia and Jack are a middle-aged couple who have learned to deal with Sylvia's seasonal changes over 20 years of marriage. Their sex life suffers in the winter, when Sylvia just wants to be left alone. She retires to bed before Jack does, and by the time he gets there, she's asleep. He has learned to let her sleep at those times because, as she puts it, "I wouldn't be much fun if he woke me up." For the rest of the year, the couple enjoys an active and satisfying sex life.

> *People with SAD often just want to be left alone.*

The effect of SAD on relationships is not confined to the sexual arena. A woman who may be a social butterfly in the summer often wants no company at all in the winter. Conversations are avoided and invitations turned down. Anything that requires expending the energy involved in social contact may feel like an overwhelming demand, to be avoided if at all possible. Many people with SAD compare themselves to hibernating bears. Although this is not a scientifically sound analogy, it accurately conveys the feeling of wanting to be left alone.

As you might expect, there are considerable social costs to such behavior. Friends become annoyed. Marriages come under strain. Lovers are lost—which at the time may be experienced by the SAD sufferer as a relief, since it results in a welcome decrease in personal and sexual demands. I know many seasonal people who have consistently started relationships in spring and summer but dropped them during the winter.

Cognitive Problems

As the seasonal people you have already met in this book will testify, problems in thinking are among the most troublesome symptoms of SAD. I am sure you can remember a time when you were not thinking properly—for example, when you were very tired or have had too much to drink. That is how people with SAD often feel during the winter months. They tend to have problems thinking clearly and quickly.

It may be difficult, if not impossible, for them to summon up the information and knowledge needed for their work—or even casual conversations. They are not able to keep up with what is going on around them or what needs to be done.

A scene from Chaplin's *Modern Times* comes to mind. A factory worker is toiling away quite well on an assembly line when suddenly the conveyor belt begins to move faster. The worker tries to keep up with the increased challenge, but ultimately fails, becoming frantic along the way. This provides a wonderful vehicle for Chaplin's madcap antics. In reality, however, the feeling of having information coming at you faster than you can handle it is often overwhelming and demoralizing.

In SAD, the ability to concentrate and process information varies greatly over the course of the year. In summer it's a snap; everything goes "click, click, click" and gets done. In winter, it's a drag, with minor tasks taking on major proportions.

> *I begin to make stupid mistakes in the fall.*
> —Merrill, a 32-year-old vocational guidance counselor

These mistakes can emerge even in performing relatively simple tasks. Routine chores such as doing the shopping or cooking a meal involve several steps that need to be performed in a certain sequence. People with SAD often feel unable to focus on the task, to remember all its different parts, and to carry them out in the correct sequence. They often say, "I just can't get my act together. Simple things seem so difficult." A combination of low energy, low motivation, and, especially, difficulty in thinking impaired the ability of all the people profiled in this chapter to function at work, which was a major complaint. In children, this combination of symptoms results in school difficulties, which may be the first problem to come to a parent's attention. I discuss the effects of SAD in children and adolescents in Chapter 5.

Many business executives and professionals with SAD complain that during the winter they are unable to take the necessary steps to handle tasks. Instead, they hide behind their office doors, shuffling papers around on their desks, creating the appearance of getting work done. Secretaries and assistants, who aren't fortunate enough to have personal offices in which to hide, often call in sick and say they have the flu, a more acceptable excuse than depression.

Tasks involving logic are often especially difficult, but some people complain of difficulties even in estimating distances. One woman reported that while driving during the winter, she had a hard time estimating how far she was from the car in front of her. A young tree surgeon with SAD failed to estimate accurately the length of a branch he was sawing off and injured himself as a result.

John Docherty, who had extensive experience treating SAD in Boston and New Hampshire, estimated the frequency of the different work-related problems encountered by his patients with SAD. In his study, they were, in order of frequency, decreased concentration, productivity, interest, and creativity; inability to complete tasks; increased interpersonal difficulties in the workplace; increased absences from work; and simply being unable to work at all. Quite a staggering list of problems.

To measure the cognitive difficulties in SAD objectively, Connie Duncan and colleagues at the NIMH recorded brain-wave pattern responses to visual stimuli in SAD sufferers and others. They showed that a facet of brain-wave response linked to the ability to attend to stimuli increased in strength in those with SAD after they were treated with light therapy. This change occurs at the same time as people begin to feel better and their ability to think improves. It should be reassuring for people with SAD to realize that their ability to think can be measured objectively and shown to change after light therapy. It helps them realize that they are suffering from a *temporary* problem with brain function during their depressed phase and that the problems that arise from their thinking difficulties are not their fault.

Mood Problems

As I mentioned earlier, many people with winter problems may experience physical changes long before any feelings of sadness occur. In fact, some people may experience only physical changes with the changing seasons and never feel depressed. These people are comparatively lucky, because the emotional aspects of depression are among the most painful experiences people can have, as shown below.

> *I am sad, but I don't know why. Life has no meaning for me—even my wife and children. I don't know why. I am just a burden to them. They would be better off without me. I feel like I have let them down, been a*

bad father. As I think, all I can see is failure. Each day I go to work, I worry, "How will I get everything done?" I often think that it would be best to end it all, but that is against my religion. There is a spot on the freeway that I often think would be a good place for a "Catholic suicide," where it might look like an accident, so my family would not have to feel ashamed of me.

—John, a 50-year-old engineer

John's feelings are common among severely depressed people. His thoughts—that he is a failure as a father, husband, and worker—are not shared by his children, his wife, and his supervisor, all of whom regard him as caring, devoted, and hardworking. They are distortions of reality, though they certainly feel real to him. In Chapter 9 on cognitive-behavioral therapy for depression, you will learn how such distortions in thinking can be challenged successfully, resulting in improved mood.

> *A person with diabetes knows that his pancreas is disordered, and that's not so hard to understand. But when you're depressed, your mind and heart and soul are disordered—everything that makes you a human being—and that's not so simple to understand, especially when you are in the middle of it.*
>
> **—A college student in her late 20s**

The anxiety that John reports often occurs in depression, and treatment often helps it, as well as the sadness. Sometimes the unpleasant feelings that depressed people experience are directed outward to others. People with SAD often recognize that they are being snappy, irritable, and unpleasant toward others but are unable to restrain themselves. It is important for the friends and family of a person with SAD to recognize that if these behaviors are confined to the autumn and winter, they are almost certainly symptoms of the condition. This recognition helps the affected person's friends and family not to take angry or snappy comments too personally.

Depressed people—including those with SAD—often distort reality by blaming themselves unfairly. Another type of cognitive distortion that may occur involves blaming others—or one's life circumstances—for problems that are really the result of SAD. A woman might say, for example, "My marriage is going wrong because my husband is inconsiderate and too demanding," while the major reason may be that she is depressed and unable to meet his needs. Another might say, "This job is not right for me. It's causing me distress and feelings of failure." While a difficult job can aggravate the symptoms of SAD, the main cause of the problem at work may be the SAD itself. I often counsel patients not to make important decisions while they are depressed if they can possibly avoid doing so. Decisions made hastily by a depressed person are often the result of mistakenly attributing one's problems to one's life circumstances, and they are often regretted later. The best way for a depressed person to handle problematic life circumstances, either at work or at home, is to have the depression treated first and then to decide on the best course of action.

Physical Illnesses and SAD

People with SAD may suffer all sorts of physical problems during the winter months, from backaches, muscle aches, and headache to different types of infection. Many people with SAD feel as though they have suffered from the flu all winter long. We don't really know whether having SAD or being depressed actually makes you more likely to get the flu, or whether it just feels worse to be sick when you are already suffering from SAD. Fibromyalgia, a condition characterized by muscular aches and pains occurring especially in the neck and shoulder areas, typically gets more severe in the winter, is associated with sleep difficulties, and responds to treatment with antidepressants. Researchers have speculated that it may be somehow related to SAD, and it would be interesting to find out whether it responds to light therapy. The idea that the mind or brain exerts an influence on the body in general and the immune system in particular is gaining increasing acceptance in scientific circles and is an exciting new area of developing research. The possible relationship between SAD and physical afflictions has yet to be explored fully.

Premenstrual Difficulties

At least half of all menstruating women with SAD report that they have suffered from emotional and physical problems related to their periods, usually in the week before the period begins. This condition, premenstrual syndrome (PMS), also known as premenstrual dysphoric disorder (PMDD), may occur all year round, but most severely in winter. Some women have PMS only in the winter. Many say that during their premenstrual period, they feel a bit like they do when they have SAD.

Sharon is a housewife in her early 30s and the mother of two teenagers. She is aware of eating too much, craving sweets and starchy foods, gaining weight, and sleeping more during the 4 or 5 days before her menstrual period. At these times, she tends to retain fluid, and her rings feel tight on her fingers. She also has abdominal cramps. But most distressing to her and her family is her irritability during these days. She will tend to pick fights with her husband, with whom she normally gets along rather well. This was especially bad before they recognized the cyclicity of their arguments and their biological origin. Now they have learned to beware during the week before her period and have resolved to postpone all contentious discussions until after it has passed. Even her children have learned to tread carefully during those premenstrual days. Irritability is more typical of PMS than SAD, where people more commonly feel lethargic and sluggish. One woman pointed out to me in colorful terms that "My premenstrual problem is like a black cloud hanging over me; the winter problem is more like being in a blue funk—it's a condition inside of me that I walk around with."

Not every episode of PMS is necessarily the same. During some cycles, a period may arrive unexpectedly without any symptoms of PMS. Yet at other times, unpredictably, these difficulties may be rather severe. In a similar fashion, the severity of episodes of SAD may also vary from cycle to cycle, from one year to the next.

Hunger for Light

Even before any formal studies of light therapy had been performed, some patients had made a connection between light and mood. For example, one woman would routinely sit in front of her plant lights because she found she felt better there. Another would wander through brightly lit supermarkets at night, while still another would seek out the photocopying room because it was well lit. It is common for people with SAD to want to turn on all the lights in the house during the dark winter days. One middle-aged woman was nicknamed "Lights" by her husband because of this habit. For some, the wish to turn on all the lights in the house has led to arguments about the high cost of electricity from spouses who have not understood the biological nature of their partners' needs.

In their search for light, some people have instinctively chosen winter vacations in the south, year after year. Others have relocated permanently. In many instances, the people involved may not have realized how medically important it was for them to move—they may just have done so instinctively. Not all individuals with SAD have made the association between their symptoms and the amount of available environmental light. Some have reacted by lying down in darkened rooms, thereby inadvertently aggravating their symptoms. It is important to recognize that SAD is a condition where the person's behavior can have a profound effect on how he or she feels. Light-seeking behavior can do much to alleviate symptoms. Conversely, avoiding the light can make matters much worse.

Self-Treatment with Drugs: Alcohol, Caffeine, Nicotine, and Others

Stay me with flagons, comfort me with apples:
For I am sick of love.
—*Song of Songs*

Since biblical times, people have realized the mood-altering effects of food and wine. In an attempt to feel better, depressed people often resort to commonly available drugs, some of which may compound the problem. I have already discussed the use of sugar and starches as mood regulators by people with SAD, but, obviously, the effects of foods go beyond their carbohydrate content. Many people specifically crave chocolate, perhaps seeking the combination of sugar and caffeine that it contains. Others crave stews, pastas, "heavy," and "crunchy" foods. One woman with SAD actually craved broccoli in the wintertime. We cannot explain these idiosyncratic choices, but it is possible that these cravings may represent the physiological need for a particular nutrient.

Gratifying that need may result in an improved sense of well-being, if only for a short while.

Caffeine is a mood-altering drug that often appeals to people who feel sluggish, lethargic, and unable to get things accomplished. Most of us use caffeine in one form or another—as evidenced by the huge success of Starbucks and other companies organized around our love for, and addiction to, coffee and tea—and it can be an enjoyable part of the day. Although the immediate stimulant effect of caffeine can be useful, the drug can cause problems. Besides indigestion and abdominal cramps, caffeine can induce jitteriness, palpitations, and insomnia. In addition, people frequently become tolerant of its effects and may have to drink more and more to get the same result. A note of caution: If you choose to discontinue caffeine, you should do so gradually to avoid withdrawal symptoms such as lethargy, constipation, and headaches—even migraines in susceptible people. But many people drink caffeinated beverages with impunity, and for them, a few cups of tea or coffee a day may be not only enjoyable but also helpful.

> *I used to drink eight, ten, or twelve mugs—tremendous amounts of coffee—steadily all day: espresso, made by drip method. At times, the amount of coffee it took to keep me going was enough to upset my stomach.*
> —Flora, an editor in her mid-40s

Alcohol is another substance to which depressed people sometimes resort—"drowning their sorrows in drink," as the saying goes. This unhealthy habit may go hand in hand with a decrease in healthy habits. So, exercise, socializing, and constructive hobbies may be replaced by sitting in front of the TV (or at the local pub), downing one drink (or glass of wine) after another. Not surprisingly, the heavy drinking can easily become a problem in its own right. A detailed description of the potential harm of too much alcohol goes beyond the scope of this book and is well known to most of us. What is less well known, however, is that in depressed people, even small amounts of alcohol, which are easily tolerated by many people, tend to aggravate the symptoms of depression, sometimes days after the drinking has occurred. Because of this time lag, it has sometimes taken me a while to convince my patients of this relationship between their alcohol intake and the worsening of their depressive symptoms. My patients and I sometimes have had to watch the impact of drinking on their mood several times over before the pattern becomes obvious.

I have also seen people turn to marijuana in the winter. One young man—a tennis instructor greatly concerned with his physical health—takes up marijuana each winter even though he knows it's bad for his health. Even smoking cigarettes may seem more appealing in the winter. One physician in his mid-40s, who hardly needs any lectures on the harmfulness of tobacco, takes up smoking during the winter, even though he has given it up the previous spring.

In people who suffer from depression, even small amounts of alcohol can aggravate the symptoms of seasonal depression, sometimes days after consumption.

So it is that many people seek refuge from the pain of SAD in commonly available substances. Some, like pasta and cookies, may be innocuous unless eaten to great excess. Others, like alcohol, can be more destructive, creating problems that far exceed those for which they are consumed. Why some people resort to alcohol, while others resort to cookies or chocolates, is not understood at all. It may be genetically based or a result of conditioning. For example, one friend of mine recalls being comforted with sips of brandy as a child when she woke up at night feeling sick. In other families, ice cream or candy may be the standard bromide. In general, these chemical solutions don't work very well. For better remedies, see Part II on treatments for SAD.

Other Conditions That May Resemble SAD

In medicine, it is always useful to question a diagnosis—to ask, "What else could this be?" Many physical illnesses can cause lethargy and depression, which is why it is important for people who think they are suffering from SAD to be checked out by a physician. It is unusual, however, for other conditions to appear in the winter and leave in the summer, year after year. Even so, better to be on the safe side and have a physical examination and the necessary blood tests, since you could have another illness as well as SAD.

Specific illnesses that need to be considered are:

1. *Underactive thyroid function (hypothyroidism)*. In this condition, people feel sluggish and cannot tolerate the cold weather. The thyroid gland, situated centrally in the front of the neck, is responsible for producing hormones that regulate the rate of metabolism. Underactivity of the thyroid can usually be treated simply by taking thyroid hormone in the form of pills.

2. *Low blood sugar (hypoglycemia)*. People with this condition feel weak and light-headed at times, usually 1 to 2 hours after a meal. They may feel very hungry and crave sweets. This condition can usually be treated by dietary regulation. People with hypoglycemia should avoid foods containing high concentrations of sugar in forms that are rapidly absorbed into the system. Examples of these "simple" carbohydrates are candies and other very sweet things. Instead, people with this condition should eat combinations of proteins and complex carbohydrates, such as fruit and legumes.

3. *Chronic viral illnesses*. SAD symptoms can resemble those of the Epstein–Barr (E-B) virus (which is responsible for infectious mononucleosis) or even the flu, which may be most prevalent during the winter. It is not uncommon for people to feel lethargic and debilitated for some time after a bad attack of flu. Similarly, the E-B virus may cause long-term lethargy and fatigue.

Unfortunately, chronic viral illnesses are very difficult to diagnose precisely, and there are no specific treatments for them. Blood tests showing antibodies against the E-B virus simply indicate that a person has been infected in the past—not that the virus is necessarily responsible for the present symptoms. Luckily, however, most cases of chronic E-B virus infection get better with time.

Although viral conditions may masquerade as SAD, the occurrence winter after winter of typical SAD symptoms, which improve in spring and summer, points strongly to SAD. In any event, since the presence of chronic viral infections is difficult to document and there are no specific treatments for them, and since there are specific treatments for SAD, it usually makes sense to treat the problem as SAD.

4. *Chronic fatigue syndrome (CFS)*. This disabling condition is thought to occur following viral infections, at least in some cases, but its causes are poorly understood. Whatever its cause, the person is often left in a state of disabling fatigue. My colleagues and I at the NIMH surveyed a group of CFS patients for a history of seasonal varia-

tions in mood and behavior and found that they reported changes that were even less prominent than those occurring in the general population. This suggests that CFS patients suffer from a condition quite separate from SAD that troubles them all year round. It is unknown at this time whether light therapy is of any benefit whatsoever in these individuals.

It is important to note, however, that some cases of CFS have a specific basis—such as Lyme disease—and can be treated. It is therefore useful to fully explore this condition with your doctor and, together, search diligently for a cure.

SAD Plus: The Problem of Comorbidity

Although researchers have sought out "pure" cases of SAD in which problems are confined to the criteria described earlier, the real world is not usually so tidy. Having more than one psychiatric condition, which is called comorbidity, is commonplace. Often the symptoms of SAD are superimposed on top of other conditions, such as chronic depression, also known in its milder form as dysthymia; PMS (as already described); and eating disorders such as anorexia nervosa and bulimia. While it is beyond the scope of this book to go into each of these conditions in detail, it is important to look for any seasonal component to them as this may suggest that treating the SAD elements could be of some benefit. In addition, several nonseasonal psychiatric conditions (such as bulimia or nonseasonal depression) may also respond to light therapy. I deal with these issues in Part II.

As we have seen, there is a great deal of variability in the degree to which people respond to the changing seasons, even among those for whom these changes are a problem. One of the most important reasons for recognizing how seasonal you are is that it helps you understand so much about your behavior that might previously have seemed inexplicable. Another reason is that it helps you take steps to alleviate the effects that the changing seasons have on you.

All of the people described in this chapter benefited from therapy with bright light: Peggy received it in a formal treatment setting, while Neal and Angela undertook treatment on their own. Both Neal and

Angela believe that they made mistakes as a result of not having had their treatment properly supervised. Neal used the lights for too many hours each day. As a result, he felt "wired"—excessively activated and uncharacteristically irritable. Through trial and error, he finally found out how much light he needed. Angela did not realize that she should sit within a certain distance of the fixture and thus did not experience the full benefit of the light for some time.

Although the people described in this chapter are very different individuals, they are united by one particular trait—their marked physical and emotional responses to the changing seasons. Although their symptoms will sound familiar to all SAD sufferers, individual experiences are colored to a large degree by an individual's personality and life situation. The following chapter will show you how to evaluate your own seasonality and help you decide whether you might benefit from light therapy or some of the other treatments described in this book.

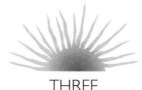

THREE

How Seasonal Are You?

"It is certainly very cold," said Peggotty.
"Everybody must feel it so."
"I feel it more than other people," said Mrs. Gummidge.
— CHARLES DICKENS, *David Copperfield*

> ◗ How severe are your seasonal symptoms?
>
> ◗ When should you seek medical advice and help?
>
> In this chapter, I will show you how to determine how seasonal you are by means of the Seasonal Pattern Assessment Questionnaire (SPAQ), which was developed for research purposes but is very easy to administer and interpret once you have the key.

M ost people are seasonal, though some are more so than others. In fact, my colleagues and I at the NIMH were astonished to find that over 90% of all those who responded to a survey we conducted in Maryland, about 39°N, reported that they felt some difference in mood, energy, or behavior with the change of seasons. Using the SPAQ, researchers have established that seasonality is actually a genetically transmitted trait and have estimated the prevalence of SAD and the winter blues in many parts of the world. (See Chapter 4.)

To understand the pattern and extent of your seasonality, complete the SPAQ, shown in Figure 1. To obtain a stable and accurate assessment, you will have to think back over a period of time—say, 3 years—when you have lived continuously in one climatic region, ideally the most recent 3 years spent in one area. (If you don't want to mark up your book, feel free to photocopy the form or download it from the book's page at *www.guilford.com*.)

How to Interpret Your Scores on the SPAQ

Question 1. What is your seasonal pattern?

Based on the analysis of many SPAQ responses, we came up with definitions for different patterns of seasonality. How you answer question 1 on the SPAQ will give you an idea of which one applies to you:

• *If you feel worst in December, January, or February, you have a winter seasonal pattern.* Almost half of all people in the northern United States report that they feel worst during the winter and can be said to have a winter pattern of seasonality. This pattern is more marked among people who live at higher latitudes. For example, a higher percentage of people dislike winter in New Hampshire (42°N) than in Sarasota, Florida (27°N). On the other hand, the closer people are to the equator, the more they dislike summer. In south Florida, for example, more people report disliking summer than winter, presumably because of the heat and humidity.

As described in Chapter 2, if you're a winter type, you probably eat more and gain weight during the winter and socialize less. In summer you eat lighter foods and relish social occasions.

• *If you feel worst in July or August, you have a summer seasonal pattern.* Interestingly, in the United States and Europe winter types are far more common, while in Japan and China, more people dislike the summer. Whether these differences are genetic or related to the greater availability of air-conditioning in warm regions in the West is unclear. If you're a summer type, you are likely to socialize least during the summer, but interestingly—unlike winter types—you may eat *less*, *lose* weight, and sleep *less* then too.

The purpose of this form is to find out how your mood and behavior change over time. Please fill in all the relevant circles. Note: We are interested in *your* experience; *not that of others* you may have observed.

1. In the following questions, fill in circles for all applicable months. This may be a single month ●, a cluster of months, ●●●, or any other grouping.

At what time of year do you . . .

	Jan Feb Mar Apr May Jun Jul Aug Sep Oct Nov Dec		
A. Feel best	○○○○○○○○○○○○	○	⎫
B. Tend to gain most weight	○○○○○○○○○○○○	○	No
C. Socialize most	○○○○○○○○○○○○	○	particular
D. Sleep least	○○○○○○○○○○○○	○	months
E. Eat most	○○○○○○○○○○○○	○	stand out
F. Lose most weight	○○○○○○○○○○○○ OR	○	as extreme
G. Socialize least	○○○○○○○○○○○○	○	on a
H. Feel worst	○○○○○○○○○○○○	○	regular
I. Eat least	○○○○○○○○○○○○	○	basis
J. Sleep most	○○○○○○○○○○○○	○	⎭

2. To what degree do the following change *with the seasons?*

(One circle only for each question.)

	0	1	2	3	4
					Extremely
	No change	Slight change	Moderate change	Marked change	marked change
A. Sleep length	○	○	○	○	○
B. Social activity	○	○	○	○	○
C. Mood (overall feeling of well-being)	○	○	○	○	○
D. Weight	○	○	○	○	○
E. Appetite	○	○	○	○	○
F. Energy level	○	○	○	○	○

FIGURE 1. Questionnaire for evaluating your degree of seasonality.

Modified from the Seasonal Pattern Assessment Questionnaire (SPAQ) of N. E. Rosenthal, G. Bradt, and T. Wehr (public domain).

Note to scholars and researchers: Over the years, many people have written to me requesting permission to use this questionnaire. The SPAQ was developed under the aegis of the NIMH, a government institution, and is therefore in the public domain and can be used freely by scholars and researchers. Notifying its authors that you plan to use this instrument in a research project is merely a courtesy.

3. If you experience changes with the seasons, do you feel that   ○ No
   these are a problem for you?   ○ Yes

	Mild	Moderate	Marked	Severe	Disabling
If yes, is this problem	○	○	○	○	○

4. By how much does your weight fluctuate during the   ○ 0–3 lbs.
   course of the year?   ○ 4–7 lbs.
                                                              ○ 8–11 lbs.
                                                              ○ 12–15 lbs.
                                                              ○ 16–20 lbs.
                                                              ○ Over 20
                                                                lbs.

5. Approximately how many hours of each 24-hour day do you sleep
   during each season? (include naps)

		Hours slept per day	Over 18 hours
○	Winter (Dec 21–Mar 20)	⓪ ① ② ③ ④ ⑤ ⑥ ⑦ ⑧ ⑨ ⑩ ⑪ ⑫ ⑬ ⑭ ⑮ ⑯ ⑰ ⑱	○
○	Spring (Mar 21–June 20)	⓪ ① ② ③ ④ ⑤ ⑥ ⑦ ⑧ ⑨ ⑩ ⑪ ⑫ ⑬ ⑭ ⑮ ⑯ ⑰ ⑱	○
○	Summer (June 21–Sept 20)	⓪ ① ② ③ ④ ⑤ ⑥ ⑦ ⑧ ⑨ ⑩ ⑪ ⑫ ⑬ ⑭ ⑮ ⑯ ⑰ ⑱	○
○	Fall (Sept 21–Dec 20)	⓪ ① ② ③ ④ ⑤ ⑥ ⑦ ⑧ ⑨ ⑩ ⑪ ⑫ ⑬ ⑭ ⑮ ⑯ ⑰ ⑱	○

6. Do you notice change in food preference during the different   ○ No
   seasons?   ○ Yes

   Please specify:

   _____

   _____

   _____

FIGURE I (cont.)

• *If you feel worst during December, January, or February and July or August, you have a summer–winter pattern.* Summer–winter types may enjoy only the spring and fall.

• *If there is no time of year when you generally feel best or worst, you have a nonseasonal pattern.* Some people report very few seasonal changes at all. These people will generally mark most of the items in question 2 as not changing with the seasons.

There are other, less common seasonal patterns. For example, some people feel worst in the spring, others in spring and fall. Note that the patterns discussed here refer to those who have been living in the northern hemisphere; the opposite months would apply to those in the southern hemisphere.

The pattern of sleeping and eating more and gaining weight in the winter is often seen even in those who do not have SAD. What distinguishes people with SAD and the winter blues from the general population is the overall seasonality score, which is greater in the first two groups than in the population at large.

Question 2. How seasonal are you?

The severity of your seasonality is determined by examining the degree to which you experience seasonal changes in sleep length, social activity, mood (overall feeling of well-being), weight, appetite, and energy level (see question 2 of the SPAQ).

To derive your overall seasonality score, add up your scores for all six items, for a possible range of 0 to 24. This overall seasonality score would be expected to vary depending on where you live. For example, the same person who has a very high seasonality score during years spent in Alaska is likely to find the score greatly reduced after living in Hawaii for several years. Likewise, successful treatment will probably reduce your overall seasonality score.

In general, the six functions measured vary seasonally most markedly in people with SAD, but also in those less severely affected and in the general population. The extent to which they vary is reflected in the overall seasonality score. Most people who do not experience seasonal problems have overall seasonality scores of 7 points or less. Most people with full-blown SAD have seasonality scores of 11 or more, while

According to a population study conducted by Siegfried Kasper and me at the NIMH, women in their late 30s tend to have the highest seasonality scores, which tend to decrease as they get older. There is less evidence that seasonality scores change with age in men.

people with the subsyndromal condition will likely have scores of 8–10. Remember, these are just rough guidelines, not hard-and-fast rules. Use these guidelines together with the other factors outlined in Table 2 to help you determine whether you may be suffering from SAD or less severe winter blues.

Question 3. Are seasonal changes a problem for you, and, if so, to what degree?

If seasonal changes are a problem for you, you may regard them as mild, moderate, marked, severe, or disabling (see question 3 of the SPAQ). Your answer to this question should be related to your overall seasonality score. The higher your score, the more likely it is that the changing seasons are a problem for you. Almost all people accepted into the NIMH programs as either SAD or subsyndromal SAD patients rated their seasonal changes as being at least a mild problem. Approximately 25% of the general population surveyed in the northern United States report the changing seasons are a problem for them. Most of these complain of winter rather than summer difficulties and could benefit by increasing their environmental light exposure during the winter months.

Questions 4–6. Does your weight, sleep, or preference in foods change with the seasons?

These questions are not taken into account for scoring purposes but are of interest to clinicians and researchers who treat SAD and may be of interest to you as well. We have found that people with SAD report sleeping an average of 2.5 hours more in winter than in summer. Corresponding figures for people with the winter blues and the general population in the northeastern United States are 1.7 hours and 0.7 hours, respectively.

In interpreting how you filled out the SPAQ, remember that the

TABLE 2. Diagnosing SAD and the Winter Blues on the Basis of the SPAQ

	SAD	Winter blues
Question 1		
Seasonal pattern: During which months do you feel worst?	Winter type (feel worst in months between December and February)	Winter type (feel worst in months between December and February)
Question 2		
Overall seasonality score: To what degree do the following change with the seasons: sleep length, social activity, mood, weight, appetite, and energy level? (Obtain score as indicated above.)	11 or more	8–10
Question 3		
If you experience changes with the seasons, do you feel that these are a problem for you? If yes, is the problem mild, moderate, marked, severe, or disabling?	Yes; moderate or greater	If score on question 2 is 8 or 9: Yes; mild or greater If score on question 2 is 10: No or Yes; mild or greater

questionnaire was developed as an instrument for population surveys as well as to screen patients in a clinical setting, but not as a diagnostic test. Therefore you should not depend on the test results alone as a guide to diagnosis. If, after completing this questionnaire, you think you may have a significant problem with the changing seasons, I encourage you to follow up by scheduling a detailed clinical evaluation. Guidelines on the following pages will help you decide when it may be appropriate to consult a doctor. First, however, use Tables 2 and 3 to evaluate whether you may have SAD or a milder version of seasonality.

TABLE 3. Clinical Guide to Distinguishing SAD from the Winter Blues

	SAD	Winter blues
Winter changes last at least 4 weeks	Yes	Yes
Regular winter problems (at least 2 consecutive years)	Yes	Yes
Interferes with functioning (work or interpersonal)	To a significant degree (productivity decreases markedly; marked loss of interest or pleasure; withdrawal from friends and family; conspicuous changes in energy, sleeping, or weight)	To a mild degree (less creative; slightly less productive; less enthusiastic about life; less enthusiastic about socializing; slight decrease in energy or bothersome weight gain)
Have seen doctor or therapist about winter problem (or others have suggested it)	Yes	No
Have felt really down or depressed in winter for at least 2 weeks	Yes	No

Using the SPAQ to Estimate Your Problem with Seasonality

In providing diagnostic guidelines based on a questionnaire, we decided on cutoff scores that include most people who have the condition in question and exclude most people who do not have the condition. The guidelines outlined in Table 2 tend to be a little on the strict side, especially for diagnosing the less severe winter blues. In other words, studies have shown that some people who do not meet SPAQ criteria for these conditions but may still have SAD or milder seasonality on interview. Those people with SAD will generally, at the very least, meet SPAQ criteria for the milder symptoms; however, they may not qualify for any diagnosis according to the SPAQ criteria. It is not unusual for self-ratings and clinician ratings to differ. If your diagnosis, based on your SPAQ responses, differs from your perception of yourself as someone with SAD or less severe seasonality, remember that the SPAQ is only a guide. Table 3, which shows how clinicians go about making the diagnoses of SAD and the winter blues, may provide you with further insight into whether you may be suffering from one of these conditions.

When to Seek Medical Advice

With awareness of seasonality constantly growing, more and more people will probably recognize that they have comparatively minor, subtle seasonal difficulties and will attempt to modify their environmental lighting to cope with them. A self-help approach is reasonable as long as symptoms are mild. Those who score 12 or more on the SPAQ or consider their seasonal problem to be at least of moderate severity, however, may well benefit from a professional's care.

You should definitely seek medical help if:

1. *Your functioning is impaired to a significant degree.* For example, if you develop problems at work that are marked enough for others to notice, such as:

- Difficulty getting to work on time on a regular basis
- Marked reduction in your ability to think and concentrate so that you make frequent errors or take much longer than normal to finish a task
- Difficulty completing tasks that you could previously manage
- An irritable attitude toward supervisors, clients, or colleagues

Be sure to catch the problem before your supervisors or clients do and turn it around promptly by getting appropriate help.

Problems may also occur in your personal life. For example, you may feel that you want to be left alone and withdraw, causing difficulties with friends or family. Your spouse or partner may find you distant and unavailable. It may be worth asking significant people in your life whether your winter difficulties interfere with their ability to feel close to you. If they do, it would pay to get help for the problem rather than risk harming important relationships.

Suspect that your ability to function is slipping if you begin to fall behind with bills and other necessary chores. SAD can cause chaos in the administrative areas of your life, which further amplifies feelings of depression and hopelessness. It often takes the whole spring to dig yourself out from under the winter mess.

2. *You experience significant feelings of depression.* This includes the following:

- Regularly feeling sad or having crying spells
- Feeling that life is not worthwhile or wishing you would not wake up in the morning
- Thinking negative thoughts about yourself—that you are a bad person, incompetent, unreliable, an impostor—which you would regard as completely off at other times of the year, and others would agree.
- Feeling guilty much of the time
- Feeling pessimistic about the future

3. *Your physical functions are markedly disturbed during the winter.* For example:

- You require several more hours of sleep per day or have great difficulty waking up in the morning.
- You would like to lie around for much of the day.
- You feel you have no control over your eating and weight.

All of these symptoms are indications that you should have the problem checked out by an appropriate professional and treated, if necessary. If your symptoms of depression are severe, *especially if you have suicidal thoughts*, you should seek out a qualified professional as a matter of urgency. On the other hand, if your symptoms are mild, you may choose to use light therapy and some of the other remedies outlined in Part II of this book.

Besides seasonal changes, some people react strongly to a variety of climatic conditions. Most people enjoy sunny days and dislike gray, cloudy days; most prefer dry to humid weather. The difference between

You need medical help if . . .

- Your functioning is impaired significantly

- You have significant feelings of depression

- You notice physical impairment during the winter, such as changes in sleep, eating habits, and energy level

- You feel like life is not worth living

seasonal types is primarily in the degree to which they dislike certain types of weather or climate. Winter types strongly prefer long, sunny days and abhor short, dark ones. Summer types, on the other hand, strongly dislike hot, bright days and greatly prefer cool weather.

Obviously, some external factors that can produce changes in mood or physical symptoms on a seasonal basis do not imply SAD. My NIMH colleague Teodor Postolache has pointed out that some people feel lethargic and depressed during the spring when the pollen count is high as a result of their allergies. In all these instances, the seasonality of a problem provides potentially valuable clues that some seasonal factors may be responsible for causing the distress or difficulty. This could even include a psychological or work-related factor. For example, an accountant may be most stressed at tax season and a landscaper during the summer. In all of these cases, the changing seasons are like some giant shape sorter, sorting out different types of people according to their specific biological or occupational vulnerabilities.

FOUR

What Causes SAD?

> ◆ Why do some people get SAD while others don't?
>
> ◆ Why are the symptoms of SAD worse at certain times than at others?
>
> ◆ What do we know about how the various treatments outlined in this book work?
>
> Having an understanding of what causes SAD and less severe forms of seasonality can help you know what to expect as your life circumstances change, make the most of available treatments, and even know whether to watch for signs of seasonality in family members, who might be helped by the same remedies you adopt.

*T*here are three keys to the development of depression in SAD:

1. Inherent vulnerability
2. Environment, specifically light deprivation
3. Stress

Inherent Vulnerability

Although SAD affects all types of people, women are most vulnerable. SAD runs in families, and most sufferers have at least one close relative with a history of depression (often SAD). An example of familial transmission is described by a woman in Tennessee who has had a long history of SAD: "We have identified [my SAD] as coming to me through my paternal grandmother, being carried by her seven sons, and showing up as active illness in the females of my generation."

In a study of thousands of twin pairs in Australia, Pamela Madden and colleagues found that seasonality is heritable. Although her sample did not include enough patients with SAD to comment on the genetic basis for SAD itself, we have since found certain genetic variations that are associated with this condition. My colleagues and I have found at least three separate genetic variants associated with SAD: two involving the neurotransmitter serotonin and one the photopigment melanopsin, which is responsible for converting light waves that strike the eye into signals that affect certain brain functions. I discuss these discoveries later in this chapter.

We really don't know why women are more vulnerable to SAD than men, but we suspect that it is related to the cyclical secretion of the female sex hormones, estrogen and progesterone. Support for this theory comes from population surveys in both adults and children. Siegfried Kasper and I, in our survey of adults in Maryland, found that women showed a greater tendency toward seasonal changes between their 20s and 40s—in other words, during their reproductive years. After menopause—when there is a profound decrease in the cyclical secretion of female sex hormones—women and men tend to experience seasonal changes that are roughly equivalent.

Female sex hormones may predispose affected individuals to seasonal changes by acting directly on certain brain centers.

In a survey of Maryland schoolchildren by Susan Swedo, myself, and colleagues at the NIMH, young girls—but not young boys—reported a marked increase in seasonal changes after puberty. There are receptors for sex hormones in the brain, and the different responses in men and women to the effects of light deprivation in winter may result from differential effects on these receptors between the genders.

Environmental Considerations

The most important environmental factor to consider when someone with SAD becomes depressed is light deprivation, in all its forms. Many people experience low energy and sadness—similar to SAD symptoms—regardless of the time of year. A change in latitude may aggravate winter light deprivation, triggering winter depressions that may not previously have been a problem. For example, a young physician who moved from Texas to New York City became depressed the following winter, quite likely as a result of light deprivation rather than from difficulties adjusting to big-city life. The following letter provides a good description of how one middle-aged woman looks back on her experiences at different latitudes:

> The last two winters have been miseries of depression for me. About February I begin to regain hope as spring approaches (in Florida), and I am truly euphoric by May. Yet even now, as I revel in July's bright days and in my own comfortable stability, I am inwardly dreading next winter.
>
> I grew up in Canada, and of course it is worse there—it depresses me even to visit there now. But even in Florida, there is a different quality to the daylight in winter: It seems as though it takes something really wonderful to make me happy during the winter, whereas in summer it takes something pretty bad to make me sad.

Population surveys conducted at different latitudes have shown that those who live farther from the equator are more likely to develop SAD. As Table 4 shows, this tendency is most apparent in the United States, where Leora Rosen, formerly at the National Institute of Justice in Washington, DC, found approximately 9% of those living in New Hampshire (42°N) report symptoms of SAD while only 1.5% of those living in southern Florida (27°N) reported similar symptoms. In other parts of the world, the relationship between latitude and frequency of SAD is looser. Although some studies in northern climes, such as Scotland, show the predictable high proportion of SAD sufferers, and

TABLE 4. Prevalence of SAD and the Winter Blues by Latitude

City/state/country	Latitude	SAD	WB	Total
Sarasota, Florida	27°	1.4	2.6	4.0
Maryland	39°	6.3	10.4	16.7
New York City	40°	4.7	12.5	17.2
Nashua, New Hampshire	42°	9.7	11.0	20.7
Fairbanks, Alaska	65°	9.2	19.1	28.3
Stockholm, Sweden	59°	3.9	13.9	17.8
Helsinki, Finland	59°	7.1	11.8	18.9
Oslo, Norway	59°	14.0	12.6	24.6
Reykjavik, Iceland	64°	3.8	7.6	11.3
Tromsö, Norway	69°	13.7	10.7	24.4
Nagoya, Japan	35°	0.9	0.8	1.7

Prevalence (% of sample)

some correspondingly southern locations such as Australia and Thailand show low frequencies, other studies do not obey this general rule. Of particular interest are the inhabitants of Iceland and Canadians of Icelandic extraction, who show a low frequency of SAD despite their northern locations, according to studies performed by Andres Magnusson, currently at the University of Iceland. This may reflect some genetic protection in these people, who evolved in the North and represent a relatively insulated gene pool. It is easy to imagine how having SAD in the North could be a significant disadvantage, resulting in a failure to thrive and reproduce over the centuries. It is also possible that there may be other ethnic differences in vulnerability to SAD. For example, low frequencies of SAD were found in Japan by Norio Ozaki, currently at the University of Nagoya, and in China by Ling Han, formerly a fellow at the NIMH.

Another cause of light deprivation, which often goes unrecognized, is a move from a brighter to a darker home. For example, a 30-year-old secretary who moved from her 20th-floor apartment, where the sun streamed in every morning, to a basement apartment suffered the effects of diminished environmental light and became depressed. Recognizing this relationship between mood and the environment, a student from Minnesota writes:

> I have often wondered over the last several years why it is that when I go home I lose all energy and have a strong desire to sleep. This occurs all year round for me, although it is more pronounced during the winter months. My house is exposed to very little direct sunlight and is quite gloomy. I have also noticed that when I go and stay at a certain friend's house that is exposed to a lot of sunlight my mood lightens drastically.

People with SAD are particularly susceptible to moving into dark places in the summer, when the prospective home may seem quite adequately illuminated and the memories of SAD may be far away. Bob Wilhelm, a professional storyteller, who suffered from SAD for many years until he discovered the nature of his condition and how to treat it, told me how he moved to the Pacific Northwest during the summer and purchased a house in the middle of a forest of evergreens. During the summer days, when he signed a contract to buy the house, the sun's rays streamed down between the trees, making the cottage seem like an ideal place for Bob and his wife. Unfortunately, he did not realize that when winter arrived, the sun would be low on the horizon and the small amount of available sunlight would be blocked by a dense screen of conifers. During the following winter Bob had such a severe depression that he identified literally and figuratively with the poet Dante, who centuries before had written about finding himself in the midst of a dark wood from which he didn't know how to escape.

Moves from a well-lit to a darker workplace can also bring on depression. One schoolteacher from Minneapolis writes:

> In many of our area schools, windows are being closed over to conserve energy, bringing the effect of winter darkness all year round. No wonder I found my classroom depressing after the windows were sheeted up; it was darker.

Even in sunnier places, however, working people are often exposed to very little bright light. For example, Dan Kripke and colleagues in sunny San Diego measured light exposure in working adults and found that on average they were exposed to only half an hour of bright light per day. In recent years, there has been a tremendous increase in the number of windowless buildings, apparently designed in response to concerns about energy conservation. Even in offices with windows, the glass is often coated with a light-absorbing substance—again, in an attempt to conserve energy. Unfortunately, electrical energy is conserved at the expense of human energy, at least in those who suffer from SAD or the winter blues.

Apart from changes in season, latitude, and indoor lighting environment, certain weather patterns, regardless of when they occur, may deprive us of light. People with SAD react like living weather vanes. After a sunny streak, all will be fine, but after a long spell of cloudy days, all will be amiss. Small inconveniences will feel like major disruptions, and there will be an abundance of symptoms, both physical and psychological. These symptoms may occur even in the summer if there has been a string of rainy days. Conversely, a clear snap in the winter may result in unseasonable remissions.

A woman who writes to me from the Northeast clearly associates light deprivation, rather than season, with her symptoms:

> *On gray or stormy days (no matter the season!), I become very depressed. The longer the duration of this weather, the lower I feel. As soon as the sun appears, my mood drastically improves. I do not like a dark environment and will seek out bright areas. Dark rooms are oppressive to me.*

I have received several letters from San Francisco, where fog abounds and obliterates the sunlight in many areas of the city. One street may be foggy, while over the next hill it may be sunny. Apparently the price of real estate depends in part on these patterns of sunlight and fog, and no wonder—given the powerful effect that light can have on mood, this is not surprising. For individuals who live and work in fog-ridden pockets, it might as well be winter all year round. One self-diagnosed "sun worshipper" wrote to me:

> *I live in the coastal region of San Francisco, where it is often foggy, overcast, and windy. I often feel depressed about the lack of sun in our area. While this depression is not strong enough to be incapacitating, it does*

make me irritable and somewhat of a "complainer." My husband simply cannot understand my feelings. When we spend a day or two in an area such as Sacramento, where the temperatures remain in the hundreds during most of the summer, I feel alive. But my husband can hardly wait to get back to San Francisco, which he and many others call a "naturally air-conditioned city." It is encouraging to find support for my theory that fog, wind, and cold can get some people down while others can thrive on it.

Light deprivation is a problem in many parts of the world. In Scandinavian countries, winter difficulties were accepted as part of the culture even before SAD was described. In Iceland, for example, the condition of *skamdegistunglindi*, or short-days depression, was mentioned in medieval epics. In Tromsö, a Norwegian city 125 miles north of the Arctic Circle, all manner of ills are blamed on the *morketiden*, or murky days—those 49 days of total darkness around the winter solstice (see Chapter 15). Light deprivation is not confined to these countries of legendary darkness, however. Though less common in sunnier places, SAD has been described in Italy, Japan, and southern hemisphere countries such as Brazil, Australia, and South Africa. Even in tropical countries where winters are sunny, there is frequently a cloudy, wet monsoon season, during which people are often light-deprived and may experience the symptoms of SAD. Even in Hawaii, which many of us think of as eternally sunny, colleagues have reported cases of SAD, especially in residents of those parts of the islands less well known to tourists, which are often covered with clouds.

An unusual cause for the emergence of SAD symptoms came to my attention when I was consulted by an engineer in his 60s, who had developed SAD 3 years earlier. It is rather unusual for a man of that age to develop SAD out of the blue, and I quizzed him about all the usual triggering factors. Had he moved north recently, changed homes or his working environment? "No," he answered. It was only toward the end of the consultation that it emerged that he had injured one eye about 4 years previously and a cataract had grown across the lens. This greatly decreased the amount of light entering the eye and had apparently pushed him over a threshold of vulnerability to SAD. I have since seen other people for whom visual problems were followed by the development of SAD symptoms.

> Researchers have shown
> that some SAD patients
> display subtle abnormali-
> ties in light processing
> that may contribute to
> their symptoms.

No studies have yet been performed on the rate of SAD among the visually impaired. Such research would certainly be worthwhile. In understanding and treating the blind we will need to take into account not only their loss of vision but also the loss of these other light-related functions.

Stress in SAD

Light deprivation is not the only environmental factor that can trigger feelings of depression in the winter. Stressful events may also contribute. For example, a young sales manager had a sales conference scheduled in January, just at a time when the extra hours of work and preparation were most difficult for him. During previous winters, he had felt quite well, experiencing only mild drops in his energy and productivity. But this time, the high level of stress and the demands of his work, coming in the middle of the winter, combined to throw him into the depths of a depression.

A young mother with SAD needed to start a stressful new job during December. Although normally a quick study, she was unable to learn the new skills that the job required, in addition to running her household and coordinating her day care arrangements. She became progressively more depressed. When she was finally able to analyze the difficulties, she realized that she would have been able to handle *all* those stresses during the summer, or *some* during the winter, but being hit by so many stresses in winter threw her for a loop.

What We Now Know
about the Biology of SAD

Although nobody knows for sure why some people get SAD, we have many clues, as knowledge has accumulated rapidly. Between that and the decoding of the human genome, it is a fair bet that within 25 years we will understand SAD as clearly and completely as we currently do, say, heart attacks. If you already know as much as you care to about brain chemistry, turn to Part II, where I discuss treatments. But gaining an understanding of the biological underpinnings of SAD—the pieces of a jigsaw puzzle as yet unfinished—will help you understand why available treatments are effective.

Are There Animal Models of SAD?

One aspect of SAD that has captured our imagination is how the symptoms of SAD resonate with the seasonal changes seen elsewhere in the animal world.

To the urban dweller, signs of seasonal change in the birds, animals, and insects around us may be subtle, muted by the distractions of a bustling city. At the onset of winter, we may see geese winging their way overhead in V formation and squirrels scurrying about to store away the last of nature's bounty for the year. The winter landscape, relatively lifeless for the most part, may yield the occasional reward—the scarlet of a cardinal on an evergreen, a bushy-tailed fox darting across a field. But for the most part, only the crows seem to thrive, their blackness blending in perfectly with the darkness of the season. And then in spring, the ebb of winter is accompanied by a return of rabbits, birds, and bugs. This urban or suburban seasonal tableau is but a dim reflection of the amazing array of changes taking place outside the bounds of the city, especially in the temperate and boreal regions of the world, where a host of species undergo their annual cycles. A few of these species offer special insights into different aspects of the study of SAD.

Lessons from Algae

Gonyaulax polyhedra is a single-celled alga that has attracted the attention of scientists in part because it is a nuisance and in part because of its physiology. It is one of the species responsible for the so-called red tides that have been observed off the west coast of the United States, where they have been responsible for food poisoning. To scientists, however, the alga has been a source of fascination because of its clear-cut daily and seasonal rhythms. Its daily rhythms appear to be governed by at least two internal clocks, one responsible for its movement through the water and another for its ability to bioluminesce—to glow in the dark. It also has a seasonal rhythm according to which it alternates between two forms, a motile creature that flits through the water during the warm summer days and the round, immobile cystic form into which it metamorphoses at the approach of winter. This capacity to turn into cysts protects *Gonyaulax* against the cold winter waters.

One reason the seasonal rhythms of *Gonyaulax* are of interest to SAD researchers is that its cycles are mediated by the hormone melatonin, a substance of widespread importance in coordinating seasonal rhythms in many species. During the long nights of winter, melatonin is produced for a long time within *Gonyaulax*, serving as the stimulus that turns the alga into its cystic form. During the shorter summer nights, on the other hand, the shorter duration of melatonin secretion turns the alga back to its motile form.

This biological system, by which the duration of day and night is translated into the duration of nocturnal melatonin secretion—which in turn induces seasonal changes in behavior—has been conserved throughout millennia of evolution. As we shall see, there has been much speculation about the potential role of melatonin in producing the symptoms of SAD.

Understanding the "Night Within"

The transition between day and night, which we experience every day, is perceived not only in relation to such external events as dawn and dusk but internally as well. People (or other animals) kept in conditions that isolate them from all outside clues about time of day will still show an alternation of sleepiness and wakefulness and all the other biological changes associated with night and day. These day-and-night states of mind, which the late famous biologist Colin Pittendrigh called "the day within" and "the night within," are part of our biological programming, determined by the body's clock. As the night expands in winter, so does "the night within" and all the biological changes associated with it—for example, sleepiness and the secretion of the hormone melatonin.

If we are to appreciate the psychological impact of winter, we must try to understand the effects of the expanding night on our minds and bodies.

Melatonin has been called the hormone of darkness because it is secreted almost exclusively during the night. The onset of melatonin secretion begins in the late evening and is influenced by the timing of dusk; its offset occurs in the morning and is influenced by the timing of dawn. The duration of melatonin secretion can therefore be used as a biological marker of our internal day and night. The body's capacity to track dawn and dusk and thus measure the duration of night and day, though long recognized to occur in animals, has only recently been shown to occur in humans as well, by Thomas Wehr at the NIMH. Inspired by a movie about primitive humans, who lived before the onset of artificial lighting, Wehr wondered about their lives. How did they sleep, and how did they feel during their waking hours?

Wehr and his colleagues set out to study this question by having volunteers spend extended periods of time on an inpatient unit at the NIMH. In an attempt to re-create the winter conditions of light and dark to which primitive humans were exposed, the researchers asked these volunteers to expose themselves to ordinary lighting conditions and go about their normal lives for 10 hours each day, but to lie in a restful state in complete darkness for the other 14 hours. They measured their sleep patterns and blood levels of melatonin and other hormones. For comparison purposes, these researchers then asked the volunteers to adhere to a summer light–dark cycle: 16 hours per day of exposure to ordinary outdoor lighting during the summer day and 8 hours per day of restful time in complete darkness. Once again, they examined sleep and hormonal measures.

When he compared the profiles of melatonin secretion in the artificial winter and summer conditions, Wehr found a pattern of seasonal change that strikingly resembled the seasonal changes seen in so many of the other species that have been studied, from the lowly single-celled *Gonyaulax* to sheep and cattle. During the long winter nights, the duration of melatonin secretion expands, whereas during the short nights of summer it contracts. One important implication of this finding is that the biological underpinnings for seasonal response—the capacity of melatonin secretion to be influenced in a predictable way by the length of the night—is intact in humans. At this time we do not know what effects, if any, these changes in duration of melatonin secretion may have on human physiology, mood, or behavior.

Wehr and I and our colleagues reached certain intriguing conclusions from a series of studies in which we extended the duration of night:

• During the winter, people with SAD undergoing their normal light–dark routine show the same type of expansion of plasma melatonin duration seen in nonseasonal volunteers kept in artificial darkness for 14 hours per day. In other words, despite the presence of artificial lighting, those with SAD appear to vary seasonally with respect to this important biological variable. Nonseasonal volunteers did not show these changes in melatonin secretion when evaluated in summer and winter in naturalistic lighting conditions.

These results have profound implications as they suggest that people with SAD do not "see" light in the same way as nonseasonal people. Although there is no evidence of any visual problems in SAD sufferers, they may have more subtle problems with processing light either at the level of the eyes or within the brain itself.

Other intriguing findings to emerge from Wehr's experiments include:

• During extended nights, sleep breaks up into two components, an early and a late one, separated by a period of wakefulness. Such first and second sleep periods were recorded in historical documents written before bright indoor lighting was widely available: the intervening period of wakefulness was known as "The Watch."

• People slept far longer on average than is the norm in our society and reported being more alert and awake during the daytime. This finding suggests that many modern people may walk around in a less wide-awake state as a result of chronic sleep deprivation. In modern times, as a result of bright indoor artificial lighting, sleep is squeezed into a single block, and we no longer experience the "crystal-clear consciousness" that our forebears enjoyed on a nightly basis in the interval between their two sleep periods. Perhaps that is one reason meditation is so helpful—including for people with SAD: it restores this state of consciousness on a daily basis (see Chapter 11 for more information about this).

> *Meditation may be helpful because it restores the state of crystal-clear consciousness that people experienced on a nightly basis when they slept long enough to have two periods of sleep with an awake interval in between.*

• During the extended darkness, there was an increased level of the hormone prolactin in the bloodstream. This hormone has been reported to increase during meditative states. It may explain why the subjects in Wehr's study were not anxious when awake in the dark—in contrast to the way insomniacs often feel—but experienced instead a peaceful stillness. Prolactin secretion may also explain the serene demeanor of certain polar animals as they rest peacefully in the frozen Arctic wilderness, patiently awaiting the return of the light. These creatures are described in more detail later.

Winter as an Energy Crisis: Lessons from Svalbard

The Northern Arctic archipelago of Svalbard or Spitzbergen must surely have one of the most inhospitable climates for sustaining life, especially among complex creatures. Located halfway between Norway and the North Pole, the islands are immersed in darkness for over 2 months of each year. All vegetation on the islands grows in the 2 months of summer, during which it is light for 24 hours a day. Foraging during the winter season is made more difficult in Svalbard because temperatures are less extreme than in other parts of the region, causing melting and refreezing, resulting in a relatively thin crust of ice, which is dangerous for animals to cross. Despite these extremely severe conditions, two species, the Svalbard reindeer and the Svalbard ptarmigan, a plump white bird, have succeeded brilliantly in colonizing the islands.

Although these species eat more during the autumn, storing extra body fat against the winter, researchers have calculated that this extra fat is quite inadequate to sustain their energy need throughout the winter of frigid temperatures and food deprivation. Instead, they rely on slowing down their activity to an extreme degree. People often comment on the apparent tameness of the reindeer or ptarmigan when approached by humans. Instead of running away, they stand still or lie in the snow and ice, staring into space. The appearance of having given up, which has been called arctic resignation, is in fact a life-saving strategy. By slowing down all movements, for example, the reindeer reduces its energy consumption to one-fourth of what it would expend if it were trotting. Such apparent tameness may have evolved because in the arctic regions, winter, with its subzero temperatures, is a far more dangerous enemy than any natural predator, and saving energy by lowered metabolism and levels of arousal is more valuable to the animal than vigilance, swift reflexes, and being ready to run off at a moment's notice. It is more adaptive to "resign" and conserve energy than to flee and squander it. It is this sort of decision—to be active or passive—the calculation of which varies with the terrain and the season, that is a key to survival in the harsh winters of the Far North.

Is SAD a Form of Human Hibernation or Arctic Resignation?

I often encounter variations of this question, usually from people who feel a strong identification with hibernating bears. The desire to be recumbent, to be a couch potato, to loll the day away, to be left alone in some dark space, inevitably brings to mind a bear in his cave. Biologists scoff at such analogies. They point out that small hibernating mammals show a marked drop in temperature that is not seen in people with SAD. Nor are SAD sufferers really like bears that while away their winter months in a sleeplike state. But these dismissals don't address what people who ask this question often really want to know: Is SAD an adaptive state that might actually be a useful energy-conserving mechanism for some people during the winter months in the same way hibernation is for bears? In other words, is it our society rather than our biology that is at fault for expecting us to function fully all year round in a manner that is contrary to the ways of nature?

It is possible that the differing historical roles of women and men in society might account for the greater levels of seasonality and SAD occurring in women. In tribal life, women stayed at home, bearing and nursing children, while men hunted for food and protected the tribe against marauders. During the winter, when food is scarce, it might have been adaptive in such tribes for women to increase their food intake and decrease their level of activity and for men not to show these seasonal changes, remaining alert and active all year long.

> *Could SAD be a way of "hibernating" to conserve energy?*

We have no good answers to these speculations at this time. It may be that certain SAD symptoms are exaggerations of adaptive responses to the changing seasons that might have conferred an advantage to an individual or to a society under certain circumstances. On the other hand, it can be argued that SAD is a maladaptive response—perhaps a breakdown in normal physiological systems—that might have been a liability even in societies beyond our own. In support of this second line of reasoning is the low prevalence of SAD in Iceland, which suggests that those with a genetic vulnerability to SAD did not reproduce as effectively as those without such genes. In addition, it has been pointed out that states of hibernation and winter energy conservation in animals are often preceded by increased eating and fat deposition in anticipation of the season of scarcity. In SAD sufferers, this overeating and weight gain generally continues throughout the winter—a pattern that would be maladaptive in times of scarcity.

When to Have Sex: Seasonal Rhythms of Reproduction

Across many species, it is a clear advantage for offspring to be born during the spring, when the weather is more hospitable and food is more freely available. Thus, depending on the gestation period of a species, conception should be timed accordingly if this is to happen. In hamsters, for example, which have a short gestation period, conception occurs optimally as the days are getting longer. For sheep, on the other hand, the optimal time for conception is during the winter, given their 4-month gestation period.

To accommodate these seasonal rhythms of fertility, nature has contrived ingenious methods of contraception in certain seasons and maximum fertility in others. These seasonal adaptations differ in males and females. For example, rams show a certain level of sexual interest in ewes all year round, whereas the ewes are entirely unresponsive to being approached sexually until autumn. At that time, influenced by the decreasing duration of the days, they go into estrus and become fertile. This is a period of sexual excitement for ewes. The ewe becomes generally nervous, and there is swelling of the vulva, the opening to the vagina. The end of a ram's penis is slender and twisted so as to be able to enter the cervix of the ewe's uterus for more effective fertilization of the ovum. The cervix of the ewe, however, is closed for most of the year except for the breeding season, and only then can it be penetrated by the ram's penis. Seasonal changes in the ram's sexual functioning are also apparent. For example, testicular weight is at its lowest level during the spring and reaches its maximum in late summer.

These changes in reproductive functioning are also mediated by the secretion of melatonin. Once again, the length of the night, via its influence on the duration of melatonin secretion, signals to the animal whether it is summer or winter and initiates a cascade of biological events that results in the seasonally appropriate reproductive behavior.

There is evidence that humans also vary seasonally in relation to their sex drive and fertility. There is a general increase in sexual interest and activity in the spring. There is also a clear-cut seasonal rhythm in births, with peaks occurring in spring, though this rhythm has become less marked over the last century as our lives have become more insulated from the effects of the seasons. These tendencies may be exaggerated in people with SAD. For example, a small percentage of women with SAD stop menstruating during the winter months but start menstruating again after receiving light therapy. Erick Turner and I reported a connection between light and reproductive functioning in a patient we treated at the NIMH. The woman, who was at the verge of menopause, developed hot flashes only during the winter. These hot flashes, which result from the falling estrogen levels that occur around menopause, disappeared following light therapy. Observations such as these suggest that light therapy can stimulate the reproductive system, possibly via its effects on melatonin, which may have certain therapeutic applications.

Growing a Winter Brain: The Chickadee

Chickadees, dressed in their black bibs and black bonnets, bustle about in easy view on the leafless branches of the yellow birches in winter. All the bird-watcher needs to do to get a closer look at them is to make a "pish, pish" sound and they dip down to the lower twigs to investigate. To obtain enough food in the barren winter landscape, they need to forage over a territory four times greater than they do in summer. They have managed to survive the deprivations of the winter season by using an ingenious biological strategy that allows them to keep track of this greater foraging territory and to remember where they have stored their food caches—they grow more brain cells. Research by Fernando Nottebaum of Rockefeller University found that in black-capped chickadees the hippocampus, a part of the brain believed to be involved in memory and spatial learning, grows each October.

It is exciting to contemplate the adult brain not as rigid and unchanging but as capable of continued growth under certain circumstances. To what extent these observations may apply to humans as well is unclear at this time, but there is evidence that certain neurons in the suprachiasmatic nuclei, the body's clock, which produce a substance known as vasopressin, are present in greater numbers in the winter than in the summer. Paul Schwartz, while at the NIMH, found that the size of the pituitary gland, which is located behind the eyes and is responsible for secreting a large number of hormones, varies across seasons in humans. In addition, the nature of this variation is different in men and in women. These findings from human studies suggest that there may be a certain seasonal plasticity in the adult human brain that is reminiscent of that found in chickadees.

Behold a SAD Horse: Clues to Individual Vulnerability

There is no reason to assume that diversity among individuals in their responses to winter exists only among humans. Very probably other animals show these varied responses too, and they might be easy to detect if one had a mind to look for them. I was called, for example, by Deborah Marshall, a veterinarian in Miami, Florida, about the seasonal changes in one of her favorite horses. The young gelding, Tango, was capable of managing the most complex of jumps during the summer, but in February, according to Marshall, "he just packs up. He cannot solve complex problems. His mind is in a fog. Whatever is a normal stress for him in summer becomes overwhelming in winter. He can't handle jumps that he would easily have managed the previous summer."

On one occasion, while Marshall was riding Tango during the winter months, the horse threw her and she was seriously injured. Sadly, she contemplated putting him down until she remembered that she had experienced similar seasonal difficulties with his mother, a dearly beloved 28-year-old mare, who would become very erratic and aggressive in late winter.

The similarity between the seasonal difficulties experienced by both mother and foal led Marshall to consider the possibility that Tango might have inherited from his mother an equine form of SAD. Horses are known to breed during the long days. Their reproductive capacity shuts down in November and reawakens again in the spring. Marshall consulted me about Tango, and we decided to put a bright light in his stall in the morning and the evening from September through April. To Marshall's delight, this intervention improved Tango's winter difficulties "about 85%." He was able to solve complex problems for the first time during the winter and to execute several difficult jumps in sequence. "It is like riding the horse I've always dreamed of riding," Marshall says, "a horse with wings." Marshall's coworkers questioned whether there was anything wrong with the horse at all, but she knew better. Tango was, happily, a successfully treated SAD horse.

As to the old mare, she was put out to pasture after her long life of service. Since little would be asked of her in the form of jumping or other behavioral demands, she would be permitted to experience her seasonal changes without interruption.

There might be much to learn from examining animals such as Tango, especially since it is now possible to detect the genetic variation responsible for behavioral differences. Such an approach has been helpful in determining the genetic basis of circadian rhythms and might likewise be valuable to our understanding of the genetic basis of seasonality.

The Chemistry of SAD

The human brain, a 3-pound structure no larger than a cantaloupe, contains a hundred billion cells or neurons that communicate with each other by means of chemical messengers called neurotransmitters. Researchers have explored these neurotransmitter systems for possible clues to the disturbances that occur in depression in general and SAD in particular. The three neurotransmitters that have received the most attention are serotonin, dopamine, and norepinephrine. These neurotransmitters communicate with adjacent neurons by means of special receptors specific to the neurotransmitter in question.

An early Scandinavian study of the brains of people who died at different times of year found that in the hypothalamus, that portion of the brain responsible for many essential functions like eating, sleeping, and biological rhythms, levels of serotonin plummeted during the winter. That was perhaps the first clue that seasonal changes in serotonin might play a role in SAD. Since then, many other clues have followed: Here are some of them.

- The amount of serotonin in the blood coming from the brain varies directly with the amount of sunlight on that particular day.
- People with SAD show exaggerated responses to a drug that stimulates serotonin receptors.
- During the summer or after successful light therapy, this response becomes normal, suggesting that light therapy may work by influencing serotonin transmission.
- Feeding people with SAD a mixture that lowers brain serotonin reverses the beneficial effects of light therapy.
- Medications that work by influencing serotonin transmission, such as Prozac (fluoxetine), Zoloft (sertraline), Celexa (citalopram), and Lexapro (escitalopram), may help people with SAD.
- Carbohydrate-rich meals can boost levels of brain serotonin. That may be why people with SAD are so inexorably driven to gorge on sweets and starches in the winter. In the summer, when they are feeling better and when serotonin levels in the hypothalamus are higher, these cravings subside. The huge appetite for high-calorie foods in the winter leads to the predictable but unwelcome weight gain that is so common in SAD. I discuss how best to deal with that in Chapter 8.

A second important neurotransmitter that may go awry in SAD is dopamine, which is responsible for pleasurable experiences and human interactions, among many other functions. In a series of large studies conducted at many centers across North America, my colleagues and I found a very useful role for the antidepressant Wellbutrin (bupropion) XL in the prevention of SAD. This antidepressant works largely on dopamine systems, although it also influences the neurotransmitter norepinephrine. By giving patients with SAD Wellbutrin XL, 150 to 300 milligrams per day, before they developed their typical winter symptoms, we were able to prevent the onset of SAD in many cases and delay its onset in others. Other clues that dopamine systems may be involved in SAD relate to temperature regulation and to ocular functioning, which depends in part on dopamine.

There is also evidence—though less of it—that norepinephrine is involved in the development of SAD. It is important to remember, though, that these neurotransmitters often work in concert with one another and it is difficult to disentangle their individual roles. For example, the secretion of melatonin, which, as described earlier, almost certainly plays a part in the dance of chemicals responsible for SAD, is under the direct influence of norepinephrine.

How Does Light Therapy Work?

Knowing how light therapy works may improve our understanding of SAD. So far, unfortunately, there have been more theories than facts in this regard. According to the leading theories, light therapy:

- Decreases duration of melatonin secretion
- Boosts brain neurotransmitters, such as serotonin, dopamine, and norepinephrine
- Restores normal daily (circadian) rhythm functioning

Light Therapy and Melatonin Secretion

As we have seen, the duration of nocturnal melatonin secretion is of widespread importance as an informational cue about day length, season, and the appropriate seasonal response. It is therefore logical to hypothesize that the symptoms of SAD may be related to the duration of melatonin secretion and that light therapy may work by suppressing its secretion at dawn and dusk, thereby decreasing the duration. We and others have tested this theory in a number of ways and obtained mixed results. Here are some of the most important findings:

- Studies by Wehr and colleagues have shown that the duration of melatonin secretion expands at night in people with SAD but not in nonseasonal controls living in modern conditions where there is artificial light. This opens the possibility that it is the melatonin itself that triggers symptoms in SAD sufferers. An alternative explanation might be that the seasonal changes in melatonin simply reflect subsensitivity to light (either in the eyes or in the brain) in people with SAD and that melatonin secretion may not in itself be causally important.
- Blocking melatonin secretion by means of the common blood pressure medication propranolol, administered in the early morning hours, may help people with SAD, according to researcher David

Schlager at Stony Brook University. Earlier work by my colleagues and me at the NIMH found that administering a similar drug at night was less effective. These findings are in keeping with observations that light treatment used early in the morning is more effective than similar treatment used later in the day.

Light Therapy and Neurotransmitters

Light therapy may also work through its influence on the three key neurotransmitters mentioned above—serotonin, dopamine, and norepinephrine. Those interested in scholarly discussions of research into the effects of light therapy and the biological abnormalities in SAD will find relevant information in Part IV of this book (Resources).

Light Therapy and Circadian Rhythms

Alfred Lewy has long suggested that light therapy may work through its effects on daily (circadian) rhythms. To explain the observed superior effect of light therapy administered in the morning, as opposed to the evening, Lewy hypothesized that circadian rhythms were delayed (late) in people with SAD. Morning light, which is known to shift rhythms earlier, would, according to this hypothesis, correct the delayed rhythms. One problem with this theory is that light therapy in the evening is also often beneficial, albeit usually less so than morning treatments. This theory has been debated to and fro to a degree that goes beyond the scope of the book.

One novel twist to this theory is that in more recent work, Lewy and his colleagues found that administering very small amounts of melatonin in the afternoon may be helpful for people with SAD. Melatonin used in this way can also shift circadian rhythms earlier. At this time, it is too soon to say whether melatonin works for SAD and, if so, exactly how best to use it.

*   *   *

Often, the existence of many theories about how something works means we cannot be certain of any of them. That is the situation when it comes to SAD and light therapy. The good news, however, for those who suffer from this potentially serious condition is that we don't require these answers to treat SAD effectively.

In Part II, I discuss the many things that you can do to reverse the symptoms of SAD and even, believe it or not, make winter a season of joy and wonder.

FIVE

SAD in Children and Adolescents

> ▶ If you suffer from SAD or the milder winter blues, are your children likely to experience seasonality too?
>
> ▶ Does SAD in childhood and adolescence look the same as in adults?
>
> ▶ How are children and teenagers with SAD treated?
>
> ▶ Is there anything you can do to prevent a child's seasonality from causing him or her problems in adulthood?
>
> Some time ago, a woman walked into the NIMH Clinical Center and asked me if I knew of any articles on SAD in children. I said I did and wondered why she was interested. "My son asked me to stop by and find out more about the condition," she said. "He thinks he has it." She then explained that her 12-year-old son had seen a TV program on the subject and had identified with the patients. If you have SAD and are a parent, you might be wondering whether your sons or daughters are at risk for SAD too.

The woman who came into my office that day reminded me of Jason, another smart 12-year-old, who had seen both of his parents suffering from SAD and being treated with light therapy. That winter he approached his father, saying that he thought he was also suffering from SAD, since he had noticed that he was eating more candies. His father dismissed this observation with a psychological explanation— the boy was clearly identifying with his parents, and what child doesn't eat too much candy? But Jason, normally a fine student, began to have increasing difficulties with his schoolwork. One day his father, finding him dozing over his homework, asked him again what the problem was. "Dad, I think it's the winter," Jason replied. And he was right. Light therapy has since reversed the problem to a large degree.

While some children can recognize that they have a seasonal problem, many children with SAD do not understand what is wrong. Often they are not even aware that the change is internal but blame it instead on the world around them, which they experience as having turned cruel and uncaring. In their view, teachers have become excessively strict and parents unfairly demanding. Many adults similarly misperceive the source of their SAD symptoms and seek external explanations to account for the dramatic difference in the way they feel when depressed.

I first started looking for children and adolescents with SAD because about one-third of our adult patients reported winter symptoms going back to these early years. In addition, many of the adult patients reported similar symptoms in their children, which is not surprising, considering that SAD runs in families. SAD in children has many similarities to the adult form—for example, there is often a lack of energy and difficulty waking up on time in the morning and accomplishing tasks, particularly schoolwork.

> *One difference between children and adults with SAD is that children appear to show more irritability during their winter depressions than adults.*

How Common Is Childhood and Adolescent SAD?

SAD appears to be quite common in middle and high school students, according to a Maryland survey that Susan Swedo and I conducted while I was at the NIMH. We found that although SAD appears to affect only about 1% of children in the lower grades, there is a dramatic increase in the last 3 years of high school. This surge corresponds to the onset of puberty and is more pronounced in girls than in boys, suggesting that cyclical secretion of female sex hormones may be one factor in the development of the symptoms of SAD.

By the senior year of high school, approximately 5% of schoolchildren in this region report seasonal problems severe enough to qualify them as suffering from SAD, which makes the problem almost as common as it is for adults surveyed in the same geographical area. When all the schoolchildren in the United States between the ages of 9 and 17 are considered together, about 3%—about two million children and adolescents—are estimated to suffer from SAD. This makes the problem about as common as attention-deficit/hyperactivity disorder (ADHD). Yet unlike ADHD, whose behavioral symptoms and associated learning difficulties are easier to spot, the symptoms of SAD are often less conspicuous and easily missed.

In another study of seasonality in children, Mary Carskadon and Christine Acebo at Brown University surveyed the parents of children in grades 4–6 for a history of seasonal changes. They found that almost half of all parents reported some behavioral change with the seasons and, depending on how they calculated it, the proportion of children with seasonal problems ranged from 4% to 13%. They also found that, as with adults, seasonal problems are more marked the farther north you go. "Given the potential therapeutic benefit of light therapy in children with such seasonal patterns," they noted, "a careful assessment of seasonality is merited when evaluating children who present with mood and behavior problems in the winter."

How Can You Tell If a Child or Adolescent Has SAD?

You can use the Seasonal Pattern Assessment Questionnaire for Children and Adolescents (SPAQ-CA), shown in Figure 2, to assess whether a child you know meets the criteria for SAD. But remember that these criteria, like those for adults, have been used for research purposes and do not coincide fully with clinical criteria. Answers to the questionnaire can tell you whether it is worth having a child or adolescent evaluated

1. Please circle the × under the month(s) when the following happen:

	Jan	Feb	Mar	Apr	May	Jun	Jul	Aug	Sep	Oct	Nov	Dec	All the same
I have the least energy	×	×	×	×	×	×	×	×	×	×	×	×	×
I am the most irritable	×	×	×	×	×	×	×	×	×	×	×	×	×
I feel my worst	×	×	×	×	×	×	×	×	×	×	×	×	×

2. For you, do any of the following vary with the seasons? (circle the ×)

Length of sleep	×	×	×	×	×
Getting in trouble	×	×	×	×	×
Social activity	×	×	×	×	×
Substance abuse (drinking, smoking, drugs)	×	×	×	×	×
Mood	×	×	×	×	×
School performance a. Difficulty	×	×	×	×	×
b. Grades	×	×	×	×	×
Weight	×	×	×	×	×
Irritability	×	×	×	×	×
Energy level	×	×	×	×	×
Appetite	×	×	×	×	×

3. If you experience change with the seasons, do you feel this is a problem for you? Yes: _____ No: _____

If yes, is this problem (circle one):

    Not bad   Pretty bad   Very bad   So bad I have trouble functioning

FIGURE 2. Seasonal Pattern Assessment Questionnaire for Children and Adolescents (SPAQ-CA).

Adapted by S. Swedo and J. Pleeter from the SPAQ of N. E. Rosenthal, G. Bradt, and T. Wehr; public domain.

more fully for SAD, especially since the questionnaire underestimates the likelihood of seasonal problems in children and teens, but a proper diagnosis can be made only by a qualified clinician.

How to Interpret Scores on the SPAQ-CA

1. Establishing the pattern of seasonality

If the subject is suffering from winter SAD, he or she should report feeling worst during January or February on at least one of the items noted in question 1, namely "I have the least energy," "I am the most irritable," or "I feel my worst."

2. Establishing the degree of seasonality

The global seasonality score can be obtained from question 2 simply by adding up all the individual item scores. Since there are 11 items and each item score ranges from 0 to 4, the global seasonality score will range from 0 to 44 for each individual. In their school survey, Swedo and her colleagues used 21 as their cutoff score for diagnosing SAD. It is important to remember this score is somewhat arbitrary, and people with lower scores may also suffer seasonal problems. One of the problems with self-administered questionnaires such as this one is that they require accurate memory and the recognition of a seasonal pattern, which may be quite difficult to reconstruct, especially for younger children. In fact, many of the children and adolescents diagnosed as suffering from SAD at the NIMH had cutoff scores lower than 21.

3. Determining whether SAD is a problem

To make a diagnosis of SAD, researchers have required that a child rate the problem with the seasonal changes to be at least "pretty bad." Here, again, researchers are tending to be strict so as not to overdiagnose the condition. From the point of view of a concerned parent, however, it might be worth taking note if a child reports that seasonal changes are a problem at all. The child may be underestimating the degree to which these changes are a problem, and even if they are minor, they may respond favorably to a simple intervention, such as making sure the child goes outdoors for at least half an hour each day.

In summary, suspect that a child or adolescent may be suffering from SAD if you find all of the following responses on the SPAQ-CA:

- In January or February the child feels least energetic, worst, or most irritable.
- The global seasonality score is 21 or more.
- Seasonal changes are experienced as a "pretty bad" problem.

Most people with childhood SAD first come in for treatment when they are about 15 or 16, having experienced an average of six winters of symptoms. There are several reasons it takes so long for children to get diagnosed:

1. Some of the symptoms of SAD fit the stereotype of what people might expect to find in adolescence, such as lethargy, irritability, and lack of motivation. Research indicates that this stereotype is a myth and that adolescence is frequently a happy and stable time.
2. Many physicians are still unaware of SAD, especially in its childhood and adolescent forms.
3. It takes several years for a seasonal pattern to emerge, so that the reason for the first few difficult winters is quite likely to be missed.
4. Children may be less adept than adults at recognizing the seasonal pattern.
5. It is easy to attribute school difficulties to other causes, such as psychological problems.
6. As noted earlier, in contrast to children with ADHD, those suffering from SAD are often not regarded as troublesome by teachers.

> It's unfortunate that SAD often goes undetected in children for several years, because a timely diagnosis may save the young person many more years of suffering, since the condition is so eminently treatable.

These children generally sit quietly at their desks, lost in their daydreams, and often don't get the special attention that teachers reserve for "difficult children."

Telltale Signs of SAD in Children: A Guide for Parents

The single biggest clue that your child may be suffering from SAD is that he or she develops problems during the fall and winter each year. This particular point may be more important than the actual symptoms themselves, which may be atypical in children and may manifest, for example, as anxiety or school avoidance. Children with SAD often do well in school in the first few months after returning from their summer vacations and generally do not experience seasonal problems until December or January. When the problem does hit, however, its effects can be marked, and parents are frequently surprised to discover how much of a struggle schoolwork can become for a child who might have been a fine student in the early part of the semester. Adolescence is often a time when sleeping and eating habits are erratic, so reports of changes in these behaviors are less helpful in making the diagnosis of SAD than problems with concentration, schoolwork, energy, and mood. The box below lists the common signs of SAD in young people.

COMMON SYMPTOMS OF SAD IN CHILDREN AND ADOLESCENTS

- Feeling tired and washed out

- Feeling cranky and irritable

- Temper tantrums

- Difficulty concentrating and doing schoolwork. This may manifest either as slipping grades or as the need to work harder to maintain grades at preexisting levels

- Reluctance to undertake chores and other responsibilities not previously regarded as a problem

- Vague physical complaints, such as about headaches or abdominal pains

- A marked increase in cravings for "junk food"

Several children with SAD come to mind: Michael, a 12-year-old swimming champion, had swim times that invariably deteriorated during the winter and improved during the summer. Susan, an 8-year-old with long, flowing blond hair and a wistful gaze, had suffered from pronounced seasonal rhythms since infancy. Her parents noticed marked differences between her sleep length during the short summer nights, when she would wake up with the first rays of the sun, and during the long winter nights, when she would sleep for hours and hours. Her problems began in nursery school, when teachers noticed that she would withdraw from friends and be uninterested in the usual routine of daily activities during January and February. Jeannie, a 13-year-old, not only had the usual difficulties with schoolwork and social activities in the winter but also became overactive in the summer. At that time, her activity level would increase, she would need little sleep, and she would tend to be impulsive and show poor judgment. On one occasion, her father found her cavorting about on the roof, enjoying the night air, apparently unaware of the danger of falling.

What Happens When Children with SAD Grow Up?

To answer this question, Jay Giedd, a fellow psychiatric researcher at the NIMH, and I followed up six of the first children who had been diagnosed as suffering from SAD in our research program an average of approximately 7 years earlier. Interestingly, all reported a pattern of continued winter difficulties. They also continued to experience beneficial effects when they enhanced their environmental lighting during the winter, either with light therapy or by spending extra time outdoors. When they forgot to seek out additional environmental light in winter, however, their symptoms returned. A few of these young people had been treated with Prozac in addition to light therapy, which suggests that, just as with adults, light therapy alone is sometimes insufficient.

Treating SAD in Children and Adolescents

Susan Swedo and I at the NIMH, together with Martin Teicher and Carol Glod at McLean Hospital in Massachusetts, set out to study systematically whether a combination of two treatments that have been found to be helpful in adults with SAD would also be beneficial for younger people with this disorder. The two treatments, light therapy and dawn simulation, are described in greater detail in Part II.

In our study, we found that a 2-hour artificial dawn stimulus combined with 1 hour of bright light therapy in the afternoon was better than a control treatment in reversing the symptoms of SAD. Because young children's eyes are sensitive to light, we used less intense light sources (2,500 lux) for children 8 years or younger but treated those children who were 9 years or older with light of the same intensity (10,000 lux) as is generally used for treating adults.

College Freshmen: A Population at Risk

Jackie's story is a familiar one; I can think of several others like hers. She was an upbeat young woman, a good student in high school with many friends and varied hobbies and activities. Although she suffered from asthma, that condition was well controlled by medications, which she took regularly. In retrospect, winters were somewhat difficult for her, but not to the degree that they would interfere with her participation in sports, her social life, or her grades. That all changed when she went to college in New England. The beginning of the first semester went well. She enrolled in several difficult classes, participated fully in college life, and continued to thrive until December. Returning to school after the Thanksgiving break, she began to have trouble waking up in time for her morning classes and fell behind in her studies. She felt exhausted in the early evening and was unable to turn in her papers on time or to prepare for examinations.

For Jackie, failure was a new experience, and it caused her to question all the assumptions she had previously made about herself, namely, that she was a competent, successful, and popular person. Could it have been that she had fooled herself and everybody else all through high school? she wondered. Now that she was in the real world, life was showing her up for what she was, a second-rate mediocrity and an impostor. She lay around in bed a good part of the day and neglected many aspects of her life, including regular visits to the health center to have her asthma monitored. When her medications ran out, she didn't refill them, became physically ill, and had to drop out of school.

A careful history revealed that her SAD had been the leading edge of the problem. After receiving appropriate treatment for it (light therapy, psychotherapy, and antidepressant medications), she returned to school in the spring, when she did very well. During the summer, she caught up on the work she had missed the previous winter and entered the fall semester armed with extensive knowledge about SAD, a referral to a knowledgeable psychiatrist close to her college, and a game plan for managing the fall and winter quarters. This game plan included the following elements: (1) a light schedule of relatively easy courses, none of which required early-morning classes; (2) a light box, which she planned to use regularly; (3) a dawn simulator to help her wake up in the morning; (4) plans to exercise outdoors regularly during the daylight hours; and (5) regular scheduled sessions with her psychiatrist.

Jackie did well until mid-January, when her SAD became problematic despite all these preventive measures. At that time, her psychiatrist put her on an antidepressant (see Chapter 10), which she continued to take until the end of March. Although it would be an exaggeration to say that she actually enjoyed the winter, Jackie felt well throughout the semester, continued to take her asthma medications, had no relapse, and closed out the year with a feeling of accomplishment and a fine grade-point average.

Jackie's story illustrates several points that are important to bear in mind in planning for college freshmen who have a history of problematic seasonal changes. First, the move to college often involves a change of latitude or climate, which may enhance the tendency toward SAD. Second, when at home, a young person is often awakened and bundled off to school by parents. This makes it less likely that classes will be missed and ensures exposure to natural early-morning light. This support does not carry through to college, where the student, left to his or her own devices, may lie for hours in a dark dorm room and miss both classes and sunlight. Finally, the newly experienced demands of college often pose a much more stressful challenge to the freshman than the familiar routine of high school. While these stresses may be relatively easy to handle in fall and spring, they may prove too burdensome in winter, when the vulnerable student becomes less resourceful and resilient, and they may bring on or aggravate the symptoms of SAD. Once these symptoms emerge, they compound the problem further, which frequently leads to failure and, as in Jackie's case, to dropping out of school. Although her tendency to develop asthma was specific

to Jackie, many individuals have special needs that require extra attention, and these are often sacrificed when energy and concentration
decline in the winter months.

It is particularly important to target vulnerable individuals in high
school, since good planning can prevent predictable misfortune. I can
imagine a time not too far from now when school counselors routinely
screen high school seniors for a history of problematic seasonal changes
and counsel those at risk. Those seniors who know they are at risk may
even consider geography as one of several factors to take into account
in their choice of colleges. Once
the move to college has occurred,
continued involvement by a caring
parent can make all the difference.
For example, I know of one caring
father who would call his son each
morning in his college dorm room.
Those short morning conversations were very helpful in several
ways. They helped the young man
wake up on time, be exposed to
his morning light, and touch base with a friendly voice from home.
Strange as it may seem, this small intervention helped stave off the
winter blues throughout the semester.

> *Seasonal adolescents are at risk
> for problems with SAD if they
> change latitude or climate upon
> entering college. For this reason,
> it's essential to address season-
> ality in high school and arrange
> some follow-up when the young
> person enters college.*

ADHD and SAD

ADHD may look like SAD in some instances, but it should not appear
regularly in fall and winter unless the child has a seasonal problem as
well. Indeed, I have encountered individuals with both problems. One
young girl I treated suffered from ADHD all year round, for which she
was treated with the stimulant Ritalin. During the winter she experienced typical symptoms of SAD, apparently inherited from her mother,
who suffered from similar problems. Thirty minutes of treatment with
bright light in the morning reversed all her symptoms and helped her
wake up and get to school on time, which had previously been a serious
problem for her.

In my experience, ADHD and SAD seem to occur together more

frequently than you would expect by chance alone, and they may be accompanied by a third problem, called delayed sleep phase syndrome, or DSPS. People who suffer from DSPS have a hard time falling asleep and waking up at conventional hours. Both DSPS and SAD respond to light therapy, administered during the morning. New research by Robert Levitan in Toronto suggests that light therapy may be helpful in the treatment of ADHD. However, stimulants and other medications are usually used as first-line treatments for this condition.

Nonseasonal depression may also occur in children and may become worse during winter. Children with this form of "double depression" may benefit from light therapy.

Treatment of Children with SAD

A crucial element in the treatment of SAD in children and adolescents is the attitude of the significant adults in a child's life. If it is difficult for adults to accept that they have psychiatric problems, it is even harder for children and adolescents, who are very eager not to seem different from their peers.

> *If young people are to accept their seasonal problems, it is helpful to present them in a nonstigmatizing way as simply a variant of the seasonal changes that affect many people and, indeed, all of the natural world.*

Treating SAD optimally requires organization, which is difficult to muster when one is tired and unfocused. The child or adolescent with SAD will therefore need the help of adults in getting organized. This can easily result in a power struggle between parent and child if the matter is not handled empathically and tactfully. It is often easier to do so if one of the parents is also seasonal, since there are many opportunities to empathize with each other and share strategies for coping. But whether the parent is seasonal or not, it is valuable to point to the diversity in nature and the many ways that different people and animals adapt to our changing world.

Depending on the nature of the child, it may be sufficient to make this point in passing. If your child has an inquiring mind, however, it may be fun and useful to engage him or her in activities involving the changing seasons and the responses they elicit in nature. You could construct a sundial in the garden, for example, and chart the annual course of the sun across the sky. Projects involving plants, insects, or animals are ideal for studying the natural effects of the seasons. For example, forcing bulbs generally involves exposing them to dark and cold conditions followed by warm and sunny ones. These conditions, presented in the midst of winter, trick a tulip or daffodil bulb into behaving as though it were spring so that it blooms early. It is easy to help a child make the connection between this simple experiment and tricking the human brain with light so that it too responds as though it were spring, even though the signs of winter are everywhere in evidence. It is even possible to study the effects of seasons on human mood and behavior. In fact, the results of the NIMH survey of schoolchildren mentioned earlier resulted from a school science project developed by a talented high school senior.

Once the presence of SAD is accepted, destigmatized, and regarded as a manageable fact of life, and once the child is recruited as a collaborator in the treatment process rather than the object of it, all specific suggestions become much easier to implement. Suggested methods for treating young people with SAD are listed below, and you'll find that they are not in principle different from those outlined in Part II.

Specific ways to help children and teenagers with SAD include . . .

- Helping the child wake up in the morning.

- Ensuring that he or she is exposed to sufficient light, either natural or artificial.

- Helping the child manage stress.

- Reminding the child that many of the difficulties encountered are a result of the seasonal problem rather than signs of failure—that it is not the child's fault.

- Encouraging the child through the difficult months.

- Getting the child psychotherapy or antidepressants when the other interventions are insufficient.

A knowledgeable and sympathetic psychiatrist or other therapist can be invaluable in helping you and your child negotiate the difficult winter months and should be involved in an ongoing way if the problem does not respond to simple self-help measures. In addition, a psychiatrist should certainly be consulted before any medications are initiated.

Waking up in the morning is generally the first battle of the day for a child or adolescent with SAD (as it is for many adults). This will be much easier if the child wakes up in the light. A bright bedside lamp, set up with a timer, can be helpful. Although a more expensive and sophisticated dawn simulator such as the Rise and Shine Light or the SunRise Clock (see pp. 154–155), which provides a more graduated artificial dawn, may be superior and is almost certainly more pleasant than having a light go on at full intensity first thing in the morning, a scientific comparison between sudden versus gradual light exposures has not yet been undertaken. A radio alarm clock may also be very useful. By helping to wake the child up, this will result in earlier exposure to the light of morning, either real or artificial. It may work best if the child assumes responsibility for waking up, because struggles between parent and child around this issue can start the day off on a bad note. I have seen many instances, however, when parent and child collaborate in getting morning light.

A child with SAD either may have his or her own light box or may share a light box with other members of the family. I recall a mother and daughter, both of whom suffered from SAD, who would enjoy sitting and talking together by their light box each morning. As with adults, light treatment can be administered to good effect either in the morning or in the evening and in conjunction with homework or other sedentary tasks. Often, though, it is a better strategy not to let light therapy become associated in the child's mind with unpleasant chores. Instead, compliance is often better if the child is allowed to play video games or engage in some other favorite activity while sitting in front of the lights.

Since childhood and adolescent SAD is a more recently recognized and studied entity than adult SAD, there is less research on the use of light in children. My experience suggests that children may need shorter treatment sessions than adults—perhaps as little as 10 to 15 minutes per day. It is particularly important that the light source emit as little ultraviolet light as possible, since a child's lens is less effective at filtering out these potentially harmful wavelengths than the lens of an adult. As far as we know, conventional light fixtures, used under the supervision of a professional, are quite safe. More information about the best types of lights to use and the potential long-term effects of bright light is provided in Chapter 7. Besides formal light therapy, children should be encouraged to spend at least a half hour a day outdoors so they can derive the benefit of natural light as well. It may also be useful to enhance the lighting in a child's room in an informal way (see pp. 156–158).

Activities that the child with SAD handles easily in summer and fall often become burdensome in the dark months. Gentle assistance with organizing schedules and anticipating and managing stress is often necessary at those times. A child with SAD might consider leaving demanding and time-consuming extracurricular activities, such as participating in a school play or working on the school newspaper, to the spring and fall months. Sporting activities, on the other hand, can relieve the symptoms of SAD since they combine aerobic exercise, which may be useful in itself, with exposure to outdoor light. Tasks associated with deadlines should be anticipated well in advance and tackled as early as possible to prevent last-minute crises.

Just sitting down with your child and reviewing his or her schedule can be supportive and serve as an early warning system for potential trouble down the road.

A review of Part II will provide further insights and tips for helping your child. Remember, you may be working against resistance. Your child may not want to think that he or she is suffering from an illness, so tact and creativity will help in broaching the topic. On the other hand, your child may already know that there is a problem. Recognizing it, giving it a name, and outlining practical solutions will generally be appreciated. By setting an example in this way, you are instilling in your child the capacity to take charge of the problem and overcome it—a skill that will be invaluable in the years to come.

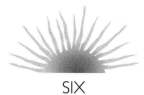

SIX

"Summer SAD" and Other
Seasonal Afflictions

Of natures, some are well- or ill-adapted for summer,
and some for winter.

—HIPPOCRATES

> ▶ What other kinds of mood problems can occur with the changing seasons?
>
> ▶ Do some people get manic at certain times of the year?
>
> ▶ What about "ill winds that bring nobody any good"?
>
> These are some of the questions I will try to answer in this chapter.

The Summertime Blues

Although the most common form of recurrent seasonal depression in northern countries is the winter pattern of SAD, it is by no means the only one. In response to the first newspaper articles on SAD, approximately 1 in 20 people with seasonal depressions mentioned a pattern of mood change just the opposite of those that had been described in the articles. They regularly became depressed each summer and felt better when fall arrived. In our NIMH survey of seasonal changes in Maryland, we found about five cases of winter SAD for every case of summer SAD. As discussed earlier in this book, most people in the northern United States dislike winter more than summer, but the pattern reverses when you look as far south as Florida. And, interestingly, in Japan and China more people report having problems with summer.

Thomas Wehr and I have studied several patients with summer SAD. One of Wehr's original patients with summer SAD, Marge, was a retired government administrator in her mid-60s when she came to the NIMH for help. She had suffered from regular bouts of depression for the previous 45 years but had not recognized that her moodiness, lethargy, and irritability were out of the ordinary until the last 15 years. For her, summers were always the worst times, except once when she went on vacation with her family for a few weeks to the Finger Lakes in upper New York State. She recalls swimming two or three times a day "in that deep, dark, cold water. After a few days of that, my mood lifted, and that summer, at least, the depression never came back."

Although she knew her depressions were related to summer, she was never really sure why. Perhaps, she thought, it was related to being on vacation. During the summer she was "too down and lethargic" to think about it, "and when fall came, I felt so much better I didn't bother because I had so many other things to do. When it goes away, you don't expect it to come back. But it always comes back in the spring." When she first saw Dr. Wehr in the summer, she said that her depression had remitted spontaneously a day or two before the consultation. This coincided with an unusual front of cold air that had moved into the Washington, DC, area, replacing the typical sweltering, humid summer days with cool and pleasant ones.

Wehr postulated that the heat of the summer might have triggered Marge's depressions and that the cool air and swims in the cold, spring-fed lakes of the North might have helped her mood. Temperature changes, Wehr observed, have been suggested as a cause of depression since the time of Aristotle. On the basis of this hypothesis, Wehr suggested that Marge stay in her air-conditioned apartment for a week and avoid the summer heat completely. She followed his suggestion and showed a markedly positive response.

As often happens in clinical work, it took a very interesting, prototypical patient to make researchers wonder exactly what caused these recurrent summer depressions. Marge played this role for summer SAD. Following her successful treatment, journalist Sandy Rovner ran an article in the *Washington Post* in which she described the summer version of SAD and mentioned that a new research program at the NIMH was looking into the condition. Many people responded.

In general, people with summer SAD resemble their winter counterparts in many ways. Most are women, who complain of having low energy. Many report no actual mood changes but feel like they are "in a holding pattern." They want to be left alone. As one person put it, "I'm just not running on all cylinders." As with people with winter depression, those with summer depression have many relatives with a history of mood problems.

In contrast to people with winter SAD, who tend to eat more and crave sweets and starches during depressions, summer sufferers tend to eat less and lose weight. These differences have also been reported by two Australian researchers, Philip Boyce and Gordon Parker, who sent out questionnaires to those responding to an article in a women's magazine and also received responses from people with both winter and summer SAD. Whereas people with winter SAD feel physically slowed down when depressed, those with summer SAD are often agitated. In addition, people with summer SAD report more suicidal ideas than their winter counterparts and may be at greater risk for harming themselves or taking their own lives. This is in keeping with studies that show that the peak time for suicide in the general population is the spring and early summer, not winter.

People with summer depression often ascribe their symptoms to heat, whereas those with winter depression more often attribute their symptoms to a lack of light—although some believe that cold also plays a role. It is, of course, possible that some summer depressions may be triggered by the intense light, rather than the heat, of summer. One of my patients with summer SAD, a woman in her late 30s, experienced one of her typical "summer" depressions after a heavy snowstorm. Although temperatures were below freezing outside, we speculated that the bright light reflected off the snow might have triggered the unseasonable onset of her summer-type depression. During the summers, the same person says that the intense light "cuts through me like a knife."

Depression in Both Summer and Winter

Curiously, some people report having both regular summer and winter depressions. For these people spring and fall are the only times when they feel good. Flora, for example, an editor in her mid-40s, recalls winter depressions since age 16, which last "from Thanksgiving until the daffodils begin to bloom in April." It's only in the last 15 years that she has become aware of having summer depressions. Before then, she lived in upstate New York, where temperatures do not often go above 85°F to 90°F—the point at which she has observed that she begins to feel "slowed down and stupid and forgetful and depressed." Her summer depressions usually last from the middle of June until the middle of September. She has become aware of this because, as a keen gardener, she has noticed that "I garden pretty seriously through June. Then I look up in September, and the garden is full of weeds." In her professional life, she is least proud of the editing she does in the summer.

Flora has noticed many similarities between her summer and winter depressions. She feels lethargic, needs more sleep, craves candy bars, and gains weight in both seasons. She has used light treatment for several winters but has not yet been treated for her summer depressions. One difference between the two types of depression that Flora has noted is the rapidity and ease with which they can be reversed. "During my summer depression, I feel better instantly if I go north. In the winter, on the other hand, if I am separated from my lights, it takes me several days to feel better again after I return to them."

The winter depressions tend to be longer and deeper for Flora. In the summer, she says, "I never get so far from reality that I lose track of how it actually is. I can't always deal with it at that moment, but I don't think that I get really buffaloed, while in the winter I think I actually lose touch with reality; I begin to get kind of paranoid."

One big problem for people with both summer and winter depressions is that they have to cram as much as possible into the spring and fall. Flora notes that because of her depressions, "I go through cycles of letting things slide, and then, when I feel better, I scurry around, pay my income taxes and bills, clean my basement and weed my garden, make new friends, and start a whole bunch of projects."

Gary is another person who has suffered both winter and summer depressions since he was 10 years old. A tree surgeon in his early

30s, he loves outdoor activities, particularly rock climbing. In spring and fall he is lean and fit and strong, "like a horse let out of a starting gate." But when winter comes along, he gains up to 30 pounds and feels slowed down and sluggish. "I can't fight it. It's as if a switch has been thrown. Each time you think you've conquered the beast, the depression starts again." Summer sets him back in just the same way, derailing his plans, frustrating the hopes that come with the spring. "You think, 'Look how far I've come since winter.' Friends come up and tell me how good my body is looking. And I can feel it. I'm stronger and fitter. Projecting the curve up, I think of how well I can do if it just keeps going that way. Unfortunately, that's usually exactly the time when I begin to get depressed again." Gary has responded very well to light therapy during the winter. In summer, his depressions have been successfully prevented by his taking Prozac. Because of his outdoor work, it is impossible for him to avoid the intense heat of a Washington summer.

Rarer Variations in Seasonality

Although most people with SAD retain the same "worst season" throughout their lives, some experience a shift in their seasonal problems and preferences over time.

People with regular spring depressions seem to be quite rare. One such person whom I have treated did not respond to light therapy but did well when given antidepressant medications. In people with spring depressions the potential role of pollen allergies should be borne in mind. Treatment with antihistamines or other anti-allergy medications may help.

Treatment of Summer Depressions

At this time, no specific physical treatments for summer depression have been developed properly. Researchers have considered trying to keep people cool or to restrict their levels of environmental light. While some individuals, like Marge, mentioned earlier, find that traveling to cooler climates, swimming in cool water, and staying in air-conditioned rooms alleviate their symptoms, others find such measures either impractical or ineffective. One colleague has had success recommending regular cool baths as opposed to showers, as he thinks they cool people down more effectively. This is reminiscent of a 19th-century antidepressant method used in France called the *bain de surprise*, in which the patient was plunged unannounced into a tub of cold water. While lowering someone's temperature may help, I do not recommend startling anyone this way. Regular aerobic exercise can be helpful for summer SAD as for other types of recurrent depressions. The value of nonpharmacological approaches, administered either individually or in combination, has yet to be properly explored.

> *The mainstay of treatment for summer SAD remains antidepressant medications.*

My colleagues and I have had some success in treating summer-SAD patients with antidepressants. (See Chapter 10 for more information about the use of medications in treating SAD.) The trick is to treat early, at the first sign of symptoms, and to build up to adequate doses quickly. It seems easier to forestall depressions before they settle in than to reverse them after they are in full swing.

Here is an example of this strategy at work. Joan is a professional in her mid-40s, whose annual depressions typically last from March through September. So every February, we meet and I prescribe Prozac, an antidepressant that has helped her in the past. In March, I increase the dosage of Prozac and we meet at regular intervals through the summer months so that I can monitor her progress and add in extra medications as needed. In October, I begin to taper Joan's medications, and by November, she is usually off all antidepressants. Through the use of this strategy, Joan has been free of all symptoms of depression for the last 3 years without having to take antidepressants during the winter months, when she is not at risk for depression.

> *Make sure your physician checks your thyroid levels since reduced thyroid function can contribute to depressions of all sorts.*

Here is a novel strategy for treating summer SAD, which has worked brilliantly for Lori, a psychiatric researcher in her mid-50s for many summers. Lori, who suffered year after year from the typical symptoms of summer SAD, stumbled upon a highly effective treatment. She hypothesized that her summer depression might have resulted from weak or unstable circadian rhythms. It is well known that being exposed to a bright pulse of light in the early morning can strengthen and stabilize circadian rhythms.

How would she feel, Lori wondered, if she went outside very early in the morning between 5:00 and 5:30 A.M. and experienced the sunlight for a few minutes? Remarkably, the treatment worked, and has continued to do so. One way that Lori can tell that her early morning "light fix" continues to do its job is by seeing how she feels when she skips it for a few days. All her familiar and unwelcome symptoms return, but disappear as soon as she resumes her treatment.

A novel treatment for summer SAD, not yet tested in clinical studies, involves going into the sunlight for a few minutes first thing on summer mornings.

Although I have not tried this treatment yet in my own practice, I plan to do so as soon as is clinically appropriate.

The Flip Side of Depression: Spring Fever

Although many people with SAD feel normally cheerful during the summer months, it is quite common for individuals to report feeling exceptionally energetic and creative at this time. Herb Kern, the first patient with SAD to be treated at the NIMH, was particularly productive scientifically during the summer—so much so that his boss was happy to let him cruise through his less productive winter months.

Such enhanced productivity is not universal for those who develop extra energy in the summer. In some people, this acceleration goes too far and may result in major problems—bank accounts overdrawn from excessive spending, difficulties getting along with friends and colleagues, and even trouble with the law. This state is referred to clinically as mania.

An exaggerated sex drive caused by a midsummer high resulted in problems for Marie, a housewife in her 20s, who was at home with her two young children. Although she was a faithful wife under ordinary circumstances, one summer she could not resist the attentions of a carpenter who was installing bookshelves for her husband. This dalliance caused her a considerable amount of guilt until she understood that her abnormal mood state had increased her libido while at the same time decreasing her inhibitions, thereby affecting her judgment.

Others may spend large sums of money that they can ill afford on items that at other times would seem extravagant. They may show poor judgment in their driving and speed along the highway, assured that their lightning reflexes make them invulnerable to accidents. Or they may suddenly and impetuously decide to undertake some long journey for reasons that to an outsider would seem frivolous.

The degree of acceleration does not have to reach manic proportions to be considered a problem by an individual or, more commonly, by the person's partner, friends, and colleagues. Others may frequently complain about not being able to get a word in edgewise or being interrupted repeatedly during a conversation. This condition, known as hypomania, often impairs efficiency. Although hypomanic people have a great deal of energy, they have so many ideas for projects that they find it difficult to focus on any single one. As a result, their energies are scattered, their attention darts from task to task, and, fueled by grandiosity, they are often left with several unfinished projects at the end of the summer.

Kay Redfield Jamison, in her book *Touched with Fire*, shows how artists and writers are most creative in spring and fall. Perhaps they are too slowed down in winter and too revved up in summer to do their best work. (More on creativity and the seasons can be found in Chapter 16.)

Summer Highs: Scenes from a Marriage

Although Jack and Sylvia have some problems with each other when Sylvia is in her "low" winter state, her summer highs present the couple with more serious difficulties. Jack is an accountant in his middle years, and Sylvia is a housewife. The following excerpts from an interview with the two of them, conducted during the summer, illustrate some of these.

> JACK: During her lows, Sylvia really gets down. She will say, "I don't know how anyone can love me" or "I'm so slow, I hate myself." And then in the summer, when she gets in the high, she'll say, "Aren't you fortunate to have somebody with my personality?" It's just a complete reversal. I'm amazed—sometimes

the highs are more trying than the lows. A day can make a huge difference. In just one day she can come alive.

Most of our arguments come in the early spring, when she comes alive and wants to do all kinds of things. I remember going to Wolf Trap [an open-air amphitheater near Washington, DC] with some friends; she was so excited that everyone said, "Look at Sylvia, she's so high." She became the focal point of her friends because of her excessive energy. It is difficult for me because Sylvia gets after me to join in on her whirlwind of activities. Just the other day I said to her, "Look, I can't be as high as you unless I take cocaine, and I don't plan to do that." At Wolf Trap she just bounced around—it was unreal. I thought she could fly, and I think Sylvia and all her friends thought she could, too!

Jack documents many incidents that have occurred during the summer as evidence of Sylvia's hypomanic state. She spends money on projects that he regards as unnecessary but that she feels are interesting or creative. For example, she bought expensive video equipment so that her sons could learn to make films, and a pet iguana, capable of growing to a length of 8 feet. While Jack regarded the animal as a bizarre nuisance, Sylvia identified with its love for the sun. She smiles as she recalls, "When he would get out of the house and I couldn't find him, I would wait for the sun to start going down and know that he would be in that one spot in the yard where the sun was still shining."

Although they have generally been able to resolve their financial difficulties amicably, Jack actually suggested taking Sylvia's credit cards away from her during the summer on one occasion. For her, that was the last straw. She threatened to leave him, and he backed down.

They discuss their seasonal problems further:

SYLVIA: There's a kind of power struggle that goes on between us, because for six months you can just lead me anywhere, and then in the summer, I want to lead. And Jack is not the kind of person who likes a boss.

JACK: In the winter, Sylvia would be really down, and I'd feel really sorry for her and try to keep her spirits up. Then in the spring she'd almost turn on me. I almost got the feeling she didn't like the person she was in the winter, and the fact that I cared for that person in the winter was held against me in the spring. And I couldn't believe that. I think to myself, "I've done all kinds of things for you in the winter, driven you around, made excuses for you to your friends, but because you hate that Sylvia, you hate me, too."

SYLVIA: Jack's reactions to me have always worried me. I like myself in the spring and summer, but I don't think Jack really enjoys me then.

When asked how she feels about Jack's having helped her and taken care of her during the winter, Sylvia replies: "I don't like to think about it."

"Do you forget it, put it out of your mind?" I ask.

"I certainly do. I want to think about happy things," she replies.

Jack comments: "The heck with that! Next winter, I'm going to let her take care of herself."

Both Jack and Sylvia agree that she becomes short-tempered in the summer and is most likely to have run-ins with other people then. On one occasion, when Jack's mother came to visit during the month of May, she and Sylvia had an argument from which Jack says it took his mother 2 years to recover. As a result, Jack makes sure to keep the two women apart during the summer. Sylvia also has to stay away from meetings at her church then, because she is likely to monopolize them and antagonize some of the other church members with blunt and tactless remarks. She relates this with a certain amount of enjoyment and little evidence of regret.

Although Sylvia's high periods are a source of frustration for Jack, there are aspects of them—the humor, creativity, and liveliness—that he enjoys as much as she does. In the last year or two, however, Sylvia has become worn out from lack of sleep and excessive activity during her high periods. She has been reluctant to take any medications for this, and I have treated her by having her wear dark glasses during the summer days. This treatment has been quite successful, and at times she has even slept with eyeshades on so as not to wake up with the first rays of dawn.

The couple has benefited greatly from marital therapy as well, which has helped them identify the symptoms of SAD, understand that biological processes are at work, and cope with these changes. Jack sums it up: "I think we're like ships passing in the night. We're very seldom at the same level. She's either below me or above, and only momentarily do we see eye to eye."

Although hypomanic individuals often feel euphoric, as with Sylvia, hypomania may also be an extremely unpleasant or dysphoric state. As with euphoric hypomanics, people with dysphoric hypomania also feel activated, experience racing thoughts, and speak in a pressured way. But unlike their euphoric counterparts, they feel uncomfortable both physically and emotionally and long for something to bring them down from their hypomanic state. To this end, they may resort to alcohol or cigarettes in an unavailing attempt to calm themselves down. They are irritable and snappy with those they come into contact with. As a consequence, friends and family often avoid them at such times, which may cause them to feel rejected and isolated. Some people with dysphoric hypomania in spring and summer also complain of physical aches and pains.

The symptoms of hypomania may result from the impact of the rapidly increasing spring light levels on the oversensitive eyes and brain of those who have become accustomed to the low levels of environmental light typically found in winter. One young woman consulted me on a spring evening for her problems with dysphoric hypomania. Over the course of the consultation, she became increasingly agitated. I noticed that the lights in my office were very bright and suggested that we experiment by dimming them. Over the next half hour, her agitation subsided dramatically, so much so that I suggested she try treating herself with light restriction. She called me a week later and reported that happily she had become able to manage her hypomania without using the tranquilizers that she had previously needed, simply by going into a darkened room for a short period of time whenever she felt overexcited. This rapidly acting nondrug treatment with which she was able to regulate herself not only relieved her symptoms but also gave her a sense of personal mastery over them. Other ways of restricting light exposure include wearing eyeshades while asleep or installing blackout shades in the bedroom to avoid exposure to early morning light, wearing wraparound dark glasses when outdoors, and avoiding brightly lit indoor environments in the evening. If these measures don't work, effective medications are available to lessen the uncomfortable and troublesome aspects of this condition.

Light restriction—periodically going into a dark room, wearing wraparound shades when outdoors, or sleeping with eyeshades to avoid early-morning light upon waking—can ease dysphoric hypomania without medications.

Although spring and summer hypomanias may cause problems, for many people with SAD, hypomanias are joyful and creative times that do no harm and don't require treatment. They need to be watched carefully, however, because they can progress to mania.

Mania

Mania, a more florid form of hypomania, is fortunately rather uncommon in SAD. In the many hundreds of people with SAD whom I have treated over the years, I have witnessed only a handful of manic episodes. But those episodes are not easily forgotten.

Symptoms of mania include extreme disruption of sleep, increased energy level, racing thoughts, pressured speech, enhanced sex drive, an exaggerated sense of one's own importance, excessive optimism, and grandiose ideas and schemes. People with mania often have little insight into their disturbed condition and experience others as being spoilsports and party-poopers who are throwing obstacles in their path.

At first mania can be great fun, and the affected person does not want the good feelings interrupted for any reason. Yet mania can be very disruptive, resulting, for example, in reckless spending, sexual indiscretions, and other serious errors of judgment. One manic patient of mine was apprehended by state police as he walked down the median line on a busy highway, certain that he was invulnerable and that the cars would somehow magically miss him by whizzing by him on either side. On another occasion, while driving around the city in the early hours of the morning, he picked up a hitchhiker and generously gave him a ride into a very dangerous neighborhood, where he was stripped and robbed at gunpoint. Luckily, his life was spared, and he found his way through the bitterly cold winter air to a nearby police station.

Even without the occurrence of such hair-raising episodes, however, mania becomes exhausting. The lack of sleep, excessive activity, and rush of thoughts can become painful, and the feelings of elation become mixed with severe irritability and unhappiness.

The following points about mania are worth noting:

1. Mania is a clinical emergency that should be treated by a doctor without delay. We now have a number of medications with which to treat this condition, but they are most effective if administered earlier rather than later in the manic process.
2. Mania is often preceded by hypomania—so a hypomanic state has to be watched carefully to make sure that it does not progress to mania.
3. If you are vulnerable to mania, as evidenced by a history of mania or hypomania:

   • Be sure to get enough sleep; sleep deprivation fuels mania; even one or two nights of sleep loss should be flagged and brought to the attention of your doctor.
   • Be sure not to get too much light; discontinue light therapy if you feel yourself getting manic and check in with your doctor.
   • If you have been on lithium carbonate or some other mood stabilizer during the winter, do not stop it in the spring or summer. Doing so increases the likelihood of a manic episode.

4. Curiously, treating the depressive symptoms of SAD with light therapy in the winter seems to decrease the likelihood of developing mania the following spring or summer, perhaps by making certain brain receptors less sensitive to the sudden surge of light that occurs as the days get rapidly longer and brighter in springtime.

The Heat and Violence Connection

I pray thee, good Mercutio, let's retire.
The day is hot, the Capulets abroad,

And if we meet, we shall not scape a brawl,
For now, these hot days, is the mad blood stirring.
                    —SHAKESPEARE, *Romeo and Juliet*, III:1

In 1983 two leading researchers in the field, Richard Michael and Doris Zumpe, published a paper in the *American Journal of Psychiatry* called "Sexual Violence in the United States and the Role of Season," in which they analyzed seasonal variations in more than 50,000 rapes in 16 locations in the United States. They found a seasonal variation, with peak occurrences in July and August. This corresponded closely to the seasonal variation in assaults, but not to that for robberies, which peaked in November and December, or for murders, which showed no specific pattern. The timing of the maximum incidence of rape closely paralleled that of the maximum temperature values. These researchers suggested that environmental temperature might influence this seasonal variation by its effect on the secretion of certain hormones. Indeed, the male sex hormone, testosterone, has been shown to have a seasonal rhythm in humans, with a peak in the summer months, and is known to influence aggressive behavior in both humans and animals.

An outcry followed. A strongly worded essay by Stephen Jay Gould in *Discover* magazine pointed out the hazards of confusing correlation and causation and suggested the "more obvious" association between hot days and the opportunity for violence when people are out and about. Two prominent psychiatrists wrote a letter to the editor, criticizing Michael and Zumpe for making "statements that appear to embody misperceptions of the experience of sexual violence and that look narrowly at an enormously complicated interaction between biological, psychosocial, and environmental determinants of human behavior." The researchers replied that they were not disputing the importance of all sorts of factors as determinants of rape, but simply drawing attention to the potential importance of temperature, "a factor that has been ignored by science for one hundred years." Indeed, the Italian scientist Morselli wrote about the influence of temperature on the seasonal variation of violent crime in the 19th century.

Michael and Zumpe, commenting on the outcry evoked by their paper, suggested that this came from "all those who believe passionately that men and women should be in total control of their personal destinies and that, if they are not, then it is society that has perverted them." They addressed some of their critics in a follow-up study on domestic violence, a type of behavior where availability of the victim does not vary seasonally in the same way as in community violence. Once again, they found a peak incidence of crisis calls to shelters for battered women in the summer months, corresponding closely to the peak environmental temperatures. Besides the excellent work of these researchers, there is substantial scientific literature on the influence of temperature on irritability, which may in turn lead to anger, directed at someone who just happens to be in the way.

Full Moons, Air Ions, and Evil Winds

Demoniac frenzy, moping melancholy,
And moonstruck madness.
                    —MILTON, *Paradise Lost*

The wind's in the east. . . . I am always conscious of an uncomfortable sensation now and then when the wind is blowing in the east.
                    —CHARLES DICKENS, *Bleak House*

So central is the influence of the moon in the mythology of madness that it would hardly be right to omit it from this book. The word "lunacy" derives from this belief. Yet the actual evidence of its influence on human behavior and emotions is rather slim. Arnold Lieber analyzed the patterns of homicides and aggravated assaults in Dade County, Florida, and showed that they tended to cluster around the time of the full moon. Others failed to replicate this work elsewhere in the country. Charles Mirabile analyzed medical records of psychiatric patients at the Institute of Living in Hartford, Connecticut, and found a small rise in paranoid behavior around the time of the full moon. The behavioral effects of the moon—if indeed they exist—may be due to its light or its gravitational effects on body fluids. I have occasionally come across individuals who say they are strongly influenced by the phases of the moon, and have become persuaded that this is correct in some highly light-sensitive individuals. For example, some people have reported sleep disruption as a result of the full moon shining through the skylights in their bedroom.

The weather has been held to have powerful effects on human functioning since the time of Hippocrates. In his famous works, he has an entire section, "On Airs, Waters, and Places," where he outlines his beliefs on the importance of our physical environment. He emphasizes the effects of good and bad winds. In a modern text, Felix Sulsman writes at length on the effects of weather on humans. He devotes an entire section to the "medical impact of evil winds." Prominent among these are warm winds that come down from the mountains—such as the Santa Ana in California, the *foehn* in Europe, and the Chinook in Canada. These winds blow vast amounts of positively charged air particles called *positive ions*, which have been shown experimentally to induce irritability in people. Curiously, these "ill winds" are reported to cause not only irritability but also restlessness, lethargy, depression, and general debility. The *foehn* has been associated with increased rates of crime, suicide, and traffic accidents. Later on in this book I will discuss the potential therapeutic value of negative ions and how you can use special machines called negative ion generators to treat the symptoms of SAD (see Chapter 8).

I have already discussed the important effects of heat on emotions and behavior, and since these mountain winds generally raise the environmental temperature abruptly by as much as 15°C to 20°C, it is possible that many of their effects may be due to heat alone.

Those who have studied the effects of weather changes on people observe that some individuals are particularly sensitive to these changes. Goethe wrote, "It is a pity that just the excellent personalities suffer most from the adverse effects of the atmosphere." He numbered himself among that unfortunate but privileged group. It does indeed seem as though different people react differently to various weather conditions. I have seen a few people who have reported marked feelings of depression or irritability when the weather changes, particularly when a storm is about to hit.

For Ahmed, a computer scientist in his early 40s, the problem was serious enough to induce him to come from Saudi Arabia to Washington, DC, for a consultation on his problem. He noticed that just before clouds drifted across the sky, he began to feel weak and depressed. His stomach seemed bloated, and his head felt "blown up." When the weather was stable, he would feel even better than normal—exceedingly energetic and enthusiastic about life. Several members of his family reported almost identical weather-related symptoms. Unfortunately, he has never been able to pinpoint what elements in the atmosphere are responsible for his symptoms, nor has he had access to the technology that might help him reverse them. Medications have not helped his symptoms, and he continues to suffer from weather-related problems.

The effects of weather on vulnerable individuals have been a rather neglected area scientifically. Apart from the specific focus on SAD that I have already discussed, little systematic work has been done on other types of climatic influences. The literature is full of assumptions and old nostrums culled from the classics. It has been widely claimed that some people are able to predict the weather based on its effects on their minds and bodies. This phenomenon is also poorly understood, and we are little further along in our understanding of it than the author John Taylor (1580–1653), who wrote:

> Some men 'gainst Raine doe carry in their backs
> Prognosticating Aching Almanacks.
> Some by painful elbow, hip or knee
> Will shrewdly guesse what weathers like to be.

Recent research bears out Hippocrates' view that "Of natures, some are well- or ill-adapted for summer, and some for winter." Just as some people are affected adversely by the physical environment in winter—the darkness and cold—others have trouble with heat and humidity. Characteristic patterns of depression may result. The symptoms of winter SAD usually include decreased activity, overeating, oversleeping, and weight gain, whereas the symptoms of summer SAD often include loss of appetite and weight, insomnia, and agitation. It seems as though these two patterns represent extreme manifestations of physical changes seen in a large proportion of the population in these two seasons. Somehow, seasonally depressed people seem less well insulated against the effects of extreme changes in climate and are unable to function adequately in such conditions. The symptoms of depression result. Fortunately, there are many ways in which the depressed person can find relief from these symptoms. The second part of this book describes how this can be accomplished.

Feeling of Sadness When the Sun Goes Down

Some people report feeling sad at twilight when the sun goes down. One psychoanalyst recognized this symptom and called it "Hesperian depression" after the Greek goddess of the dusk, Hesperus. Some individuals with SAD complain of this problem. For example, one woman observed that she could not keep working after the sunset. Another felt unable to make love to her husband except during the day, when the sun was shining.

It's a curious symptom because it suggests an immediate response to the light. This coincides with the experience of some people who experience an increase in energy within the first half hour of light treatment.

As we have seen, many people are markedly affected by the changing seasons and weather, and these effects can disrupt their lives. The chapters that follow describe in detail what can be done to alleviate these problems.

Part II

Treatments

Everybody talks about the weather; but nobody does
anything about it.
— CHARLES DUDLEY WARNER

Although there may still be little that we can do about the
weather itself—other than to escape from it—there are many
things that we can do to alleviate the effects that the weather
has on us. Along with the initial description of SAD in 1984
came the development of light therapy. Since then light therapy has undergone many changes to make it as effective and
practical as possible. Equally exciting, however, has been
the development of other types of treatment, notably antidepressant medications, psychotherapy, and meditation, which
promise to make SAD more treatable than ever.

The detailed discussion of all these treatments in this section should enable you to evaluate what therapies might work
best for you and how best to implement them. In my experience, knowledgeable individuals make the best patients. Nevertheless, there are limits to self-help. While you may be able
to use light therapy (Chapter 7) and the measures described in
Chapter 8 largely as self-help, you will of course need profes-

sional help if you choose to pursue psychotherapy or antidepressants (Chapters 9 and 10, respectively). Even if you choose to pursue meditation, my latest recommendation for SAD, you will benefit by finding an appropriate guide or teacher. Whatever blend of treatments you prefer, remember that a competent, empathic, and open-minded physician or therapist is an invaluable guide and companion for a depressed person. Depression is a serious condition that in its most extreme forms can actually rob a person of life. Therefore, *if your symptoms are causing you a great deal of pain, if they are disrupting your physical functioning, your work, or your personal life to more than a minor degree, and certainly if you have any ideas that life is not worth living, do seek the help of a qualified physician or therapist without delay.*

It is often easy to diagnose SAD on the basis of history, but other conditions can masquerade as SAD, such as underactivity of the thyroid, hypoglycemia, chronic viral illnesses, and chronic fatigue syndrome. These problems should be considered and ruled out before SAD is diagnosed.

Remember, if the first treatment you try doesn't help, do not despair, but try other approaches as well. If a treatment doesn't work, it is possible that the treatment is not being implemented correctly. A professional may be able to detect this and make the necessary suggestions for correcting the problem. Side effects may develop, and an expert may be able to minimize these.

Even if you do have a physician or therapist, the information that follows may be useful in guiding you to recovery. I draw on many years of experience as a psychiatrist, researcher, and SAD sufferer. So read on to find out about the many things you can do to overcome SAD and feel well all year long. In addition, I have included a special chapter to provide guidance to friends and loved ones of people with SAD to help them through the dark winter months.

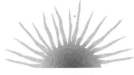

Light Therapy

> ▶ Are you likely to benefit from light therapy?
>
> ▶ How can you make light therapy work best for you?
>
> ▶ Will light therapy alone be enough to ease your symptoms?
>
> *"Mehr licht,"* exclaimed the famous German poet Goethe as he lay dying—"more light." With these words, Goethe summed up the chief principle involved in successful light therapy. Individuals with SAD develop their symptoms during the short, dark days of winter or when they are deprived of light for any reason. The basic principle involved in light therapy is to replace the light that is missing and help you feel more energetic and cheerful, more like the way you feel during the summer. In this chapter you will learn how to tap this powerful treatment for yourself.

To answer the first question above, most people with SAD do benefit from light therapy. Some people, however, do not respond despite their best efforts—or using light therapy proves too inconvenient. Fortunately, SAD can also be treated effectively without light therapy—for example, with medications or psychotherapy, as detailed in the chapters that follow. Also keep in mind that light therapy is usually only part of the solution (see Chapters 8–11 for other elements of treatment that can complement light therapy). One way or another,

most people with SAD can benefit substantially from available treatments.

There are many tricks to making light therapy work best for you,
detailed in this chapter. Reading this chapter carefully can prevent you
from buying the wrong type of light fixture or using it in the wrong
way and prematurely concluding that light therapy isn't for you.

You can bring more light into your life during the winter in many
different ways. For example, you can make a point of going outdoors
on a bright winter's day or bring more lamps into your house or work
space—both useful strategies. In practice, however, the most effective
and best-studied way of boosting your environmental light is by means
of a special light fixture or light box, the most commonly used method
for administering light therapy. Other ways of administering light therapy include the portable, head-mounted light visor and devices that
simulate a summer dawn on a winter morning. In this chapter, I will
discuss all of these, but since the light box has the longest and best-
established track record for successfully treating SAD, it is a starting
point for our discussion—and for most light therapy programs.

The Essentials of Light Therapy

After establishing that you need light therapy:

1. Obtain a suitable light box.
2. Set the light box up in a convenient place at home or at work,
   or both.
3. Sit in front of the light box for a certain amount of time (usually
   between 20 and 90 minutes each day).
4. Try to get as much of your light therapy as early in the morning
   as possible.
5. Be sure to sit in such a way that the correct amount of light falls
   on your eyes.
6. Repeat this procedure each day throughout the season of risk—
   though you may modify the amount of light needed, according
   to your level of symptoms.

Although this remedy sounds simple, in practice many questions arise about the best use of light therapy. An enormous amount

of research has been conducted on light therapy since our first studies in the early 1980s: about 60 controlled scientific studies by my latest count. A meta-analysis by Robert Golden, currently Dean of the School of Medicine at the University of Wisconsin, found that light therapy is as effective for SAD as antidepressants are for nonseasonal depression. Many light therapy studies have explored important practical questions, such as the best time of day for treatment or how bright the light should be. In addition, many different devices are now available for administering light therapy. How can you make sense of these many studies and determine what type of device might be best for you? In the section that follows I will answer the most commonly asked questions about light therapy, referring to the research wherever possible. I will also draw on my own extensive experience with this form of treatment, personally and with hundreds of patients with SAD.

Following are the most common questions that I have encountered in the many years I have been using light therapy. If you want to be fully informed, read them all—but if you want a quick reference to particular questions, see Table 5.

Questions Frequently Asked about Light Therapy

1. Should I involve a professional, or can I treat my symptoms on my own?

Ideally, anyone who undertakes light treatment for SAD should be supervised by a physician or other qualified therapist for several reasons. It is important that the diagnosis be confirmed, that a careful history be taken, and, if necessary, that a physical examination be performed. Professional input can also be very helpful in monitoring your mood and any side effects that may develop in the course of treatment. Light therapy may not work, and a professional can recommend or prescribe alternative or supplementary treatments. Above all, an informed perspective, encouragement, and support can be invaluable in guiding one through the ordeal of depression.

Practically speaking, though, a qualified professional is not always available, in which case if your symptoms are relatively mild you could undertake a time-limited trial (no more than, say, 2 weeks) of light

TABLE 5. Frequently Asked Light Therapy Questions

TABLE 5 (*cont.*)

therapy to determine whether that will take care of the problem. If it does, treatment may be continued and no outside assistance may be needed. If problems persist, however, it is certainly worth bringing a professional into the picture sooner rather than later. Guidelines as to when it is really critical to involve a professional are provided on pages 59–61 and 117–118.

2. What is a suitable light box for light therapy?

Suitable light boxes are usually metal or plastic fixtures of varying size, containing ordinary white fluorescent lightbulbs set behind plastic diffusing screens, which house a film that filters out most of the ultraviolet (UV) rays from the fluorescent bulbs. These types of light fixtures, which have been used in almost all research studies showing that light therapy is effective for SAD, have an illuminated surface that is at least about 1 foot square. The many smaller boxes on the market that have capitalized on the success of their larger counterparts are probably less effective (see also question 5 below), though this has never been systematically studied.

Some of the most effective types of light fixtures are constructed so that they can be positioned toward the eye at an angle, with the upper edge of the light source tilted forward. This setup maximizes light exposure while minimizing glare. An upright type of light box, however, is often more useful for illuminating an interior space because it projects light farther into the room. Some boxes are constructed so that they can be set up in either an upright or an angled position, thereby offering the user both choices. Three of the light fixtures that have desirable features and come from established companies are shown in Figures 3a and 3b, along with a popular smaller model (3c).

The amount of light (or intensity) found to be therapeutic ranges from 2,500 to 10,000 lux (lux is a measurement of intensity). To give you an idea of how much light this is, the average room at night is illuminated at a level of 300 to 500 lux; offices are usually somewhat brighter—between 500 and 700 lux. The amount of light coming off the sky at sunrise, just before the sun crests the horizon on a cloudless day, is about 10,000 lux year round, whereas the amount of light coming off a summer sky is over 100,000 lux.

The initial studies of light therapy for SAD used light boxes that emitted 2,500 lux, which proved to be therapeutic. More recently, the higher levels of light intensity have been preferred because they are more effective and allow for shorter daily treatments.

Fluorescent bulbs are preferable to incandescent ones because they spread the light out over a wide surface area, which is safer and probably more effective. Incandescent lamps generate a great deal of light

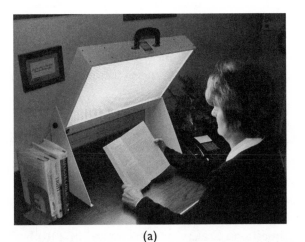

(a)

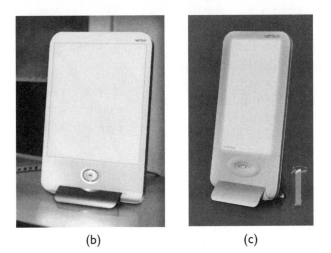

(b)   (c)

FIGURE 3. Three standard-sized light boxes are shown in panels (a) (Sun-Ray II by SunBox) and (b) (Happy Light VT-40 by Verilux), while a smaller box is shown in (c) (Happy VT-20 by Verilux).

from small point sources. These can be dangerous to stare at directly, especially the intensely bright halogen lamps. Incandescent lights are fine to use as indirect lighting to enhance the general level of indoor illumination but are not generally suitable for formal light therapy. In the United States, incandescent lights are in the process of being phased out because they are not energy efficient and give off more heat than light.

The plastic diffuser adds extra protection to the light box by further spreading the light out over the surface of the fixture. A UV filter is a valuable addition because the UV rays that emanate from fluorescent lightbulbs can be harmful to the eyes and the skin. By filtering out most of these rays, the filter minimizes these potential harmful effects of light therapy.

Some light fixtures use light-emitting diodes (LEDs)—either white or blue—which have generated considerable controversy in the lighting field. On the one hand, if these fixtures are safe and effective, they would certainly be handy, given their light weight and portability. Unfortunately, they do not have the track record of the larger fluorescent-based fixtures. Compared to the standard fixtures, there is little efficacy data for the LED-based fixtures. Of even more concern, however, is the question of safety, an issue raised in 2010 by ANSES, the French agency for food, environmental, and occupational health and safety, in regard to both white and blue LEDs. One ANSES report states simply, "The blue light necessary to obtain white light LEDs causes toxic stress to the retina." They point out that LED systems can produce "intensities of light up to 1,000 times higher than traditional lighting systems, thus creating a risk of glare" and that they can cause visual discomfort.

> *Never stare directly at LEDs or incandescent lightbulbs, especially halogens.*

Bottom line: Since there is excellent safety and efficacy data for fluorescent-based light fixtures, which have been used for treating SAD since the early 1980s, I recommend them over the newer LED-based fixtures, for which such data are lacking. Remember, the older incandescent lights can also be risky if stared at directly.

3. Where can I obtain a suitable light fixture?

In general, light fixtures fall into two categories: desk or tabletop models such as those shown in Figure 3 and a freestanding model such as that shown in Figure 4. In Part IV I list some of the established companies that sell light fixtures suitable for light therapy. All should offer 30-day, money-back guarantees if you are not satisfied with their products. (Be sure to check on this before making a purchase.) All provide details about their products without charge and will ship the desired fixture to you.

4. How much does a light box cost?

Although prices vary, over the last several years most recommended light boxes have run between $100 and $250, an amount many peo-

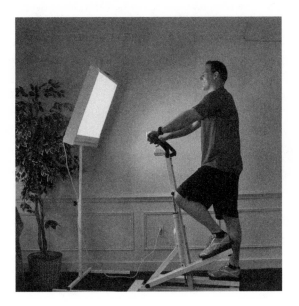

FIGURE 4. The Sun Square. This freestanding light box by the Sun-Box Company allows the user to receive light therapy in a variety of settings, including while exercising on a stationary bicycle or treadmill.

For those with more severe SAD, the Sun Square or one of the other larger boxes in Figure 3 are preferred.

Since most light box companies have a 30-day return policy and since light therapy usually works within a few weeks—if it is going to work at all—you can make use of the return policy to test whether the investment is worth your while, without any cost to you.

ple have found to be well worth the investment over time. Be sure to inquire about physician referral and other available discounts.

5. What about smaller, cheaper light boxes?

Light boxes that are smaller and cheaper than those just described are widely advertised and appear to be quite popular. If you are suffering from depression as a result of insufficient environmental light, any light fixture that increases your exposure to light may be helpful. But these smaller boxes have not been researched to the same extent as the larger boxes, and I suspect they are not as effective, for two reasons. First, they do not give out as much light as the larger boxes. Second, the amount of light to which your eyes are exposed depends on the position of your head in relation to the light box, and with a very small light box, minor movements of the head will greatly decrease the amount of light to which you are exposed. Still, if a more expensive box is out of your reach—or too big for your desk or tabletop—a smaller one (see Figure 3c) is far better than nothing. If your symptoms are generally milder—in the subsyndromal winter blues range—these smaller boxes might work perfectly well. They are popular for a reason, and many people who have used them have given favorable reports on them. If your symptoms are more severe, however—in the diagnosable SAD range—you should probably invest in one of the larger boxes (see Figures 3a, 3b, and 4).

With the growing awareness of SAD and the beneficial effects of light, manufacturers are offering a greater variety of shapes, sizes, and designs, allowing consumers to choose those elements that best match their own needs.

6. Can I build my own light box?

Perhaps you can. The structure of a light box is not that complicated. When I first began recommending light therapy in the early 1980s, there were no commercial light box vendors. I told patients what sorts of metal boxes and lightbulbs to purchase and told them to be sure to wire the boxes properly. Most found the process tedious and unappealing and were very pleased when commercial light box providers arrived on the scene.

In addition, I was never sure that a homemade box gave off sufficient light, because different boxes have different physical properties. If the depression did not lift after a few weeks of therapy, it was never clear whether the box was unsatisfactory or the patient was not a good light therapy candidate. Commercial fixtures have additional advantages over homemade products, such as a UV filter and special ballasts to decrease flicker. For a homemade version to be of comparable quality, these components would need to be included in the design. Before you go to all the trouble of making your own light box, consider all these factors. You might also want to check how much (or little) money you will save by doing so.

One cautionary tale: A colleague of mine had a patient who built his own homemade light fixture, which consisted of fluorescent lamps without a plastic diffusing screen. The patient decided to treat himself with this device by staring at the unshielded lightbulbs for extended periods and suffered a burn on his cornea as a consequence.

7. What effects might I hope for after starting light therapy?

The first sensations you experience in response to light therapy may be physical—a sense of lightening of the body, calm, or increased energy. There may be a feeling of "butterflies in the stomach" or "pins and needles" in the hands. In the days that follow, people report that it feels as though some fundamental problem is being corrected; ideally, the symptoms of SAD disappear, one by one—or all at once. In people in whom this effect takes hold completely, the results may seem dramatic, almost a miracle. In others, the result is less complete. In a small minority light treatment may not work at all. The good news is that over 80% of people with SAD or the winter blues may expect to benefit from light therapy, but you should not expect it to cure all your winter difficulties.

While on light therapy, people typically feel more energetic. Suddenly, chores and daily activities no longer feel like drudgery. Along with a physical sense of lightness, the burden of living, of carrying your body around from place to place, seems lighter, and the overwhelming need to sleep subsides. Suddenly, you feel less driven by cravings for sweets and starches. Cakes and candy bars become resistible. Even dieting seems possible again! Thinking becomes more efficient. No longer does your mind creak along like an old machine in need of oiling. Your computer is up and running again. Computations and calculations are easier, and new ideas spring readily to mind. You think of tackling problems in ways that hadn't occurred to you before. Exercise becomes less onerous—that trip to the gym, that walk, jog, aerobics class, or elliptical now seem manageable. There is once again a wish to communicate: to call friends, write e-mails, arrange trips to the movies, a ball game, or the theater. Sex seems not only possible but actually desirable. In short, you feel human again.

If you wish to monitor your progress on light therapy, consult the Daily Mood Log at the end of the book (Appendix A, p. 328), which may help you measure your mood level on a daily basis. Feel free to photocopy the form or download it from the book's page at *www.guilford.com*.

8. How long does it take for light therapy to begin to work?

Although this varies from person to person, most feel the effects of light therapy within 2 to 4 days of starting treatment. Some experience a lift in mood and energy level after only one session of light therapy. Almost everyone who is going to respond to light therapy should feel the benefit within 2 weeks, though it may be worth persevering beyond that time.

Those who experience an immediate positive effect of bright light may be the ones who experience "light hunger" during the winter and have learned to seek out bright places. On the other hand, those who respond to light therapy more slowly, over days or weeks, may be the ones who have not learned to associated their down feelings with the brightness of their environment. These people may therefore seclude themselves when they feel depressed and rest in dark rooms, thereby inadvertently making their symptoms worse.

When I think back to those who have experienced an immediate response to light therapy, the man who comes first to mind is a car salesman in his early 30s. He had suffered winter depressions for several years and had used cocaine in an attempt to increase his energy level and remain functional at his work during the winter months. It is hard to imagine a job more difficult for a depressed person than that of a salesman, whose livelihood depends on being upbeat and persuasive. Although cocaine seemed to help in the short run, over time the drug made matters much worse. He became increasingly addicted and experienced many of the problems associated with this dangerous substance. He had quit cocaine a few years previously with great difficulty, but now, confronted once again with an impending winter depression and unable to function at work, he was tempted to start using cocaine again—unless, he informed me, I could find something else to improve his mood quickly.

As he began his story, his slow, listless demeanor made it hard to imagine him selling anything—or functioning at all for that matter. I wondered what would happen if I turned on the light box in my office—so I did. Within half an hour, he showed a marked improvement as we talked. The pace of his speech picked up; life returned to his face and body gestures, and enthusiasm to his voice. At that moment, it was clear how successful a salesman he could be when he was well. He went on to use light successfully throughout the winter and did not feel any further need for cocaine.

I have since used the light box during treatment sessions with several patients with SAD who have dragged themselves into my office at the beginning of the session and have left with smiles on their faces and a spring in their stride.

Not everybody is a rapid responder, however, so don't be disappointed if you're not one of them.

> *Persevere with light treatment consistently for at least 2 weeks and, if you don't feel better, review the section on troubleshooting before concluding that light treatment is not for you (see pp. 149–150).*

9. Do I need to stare at the light box?

No. Studies show that it is not necessary to stare at the light box to derive its benefits. Just facing it with your eyes open is generally sufficient for obtaining a therapeutic effect. It is important, however, that your eyes be open. In an early NIMH study, Wehr and I found that the beneficial effects of light therapy enter via the eyes rather than the skin. It is quite safe, however—if you are using a properly made light box—to stare at the plastic diffusing screen for short periods (such as a minute or two). Because you are not obligated to stare at the light box, there are many things you can do while receiving treatment. (See question 12.)

10. Where is the light acting?

Evidence suggests that light therapy acts on the brain via connections from the eyes. (See Chapter 4 for more details.) That is why it is necessary to face the light box.

One study showing that light exposure to the back of the knees could alter the timing of daily rhythms was never replicated. There is no basis for recommending that light be used in this way.

In Finland, there are ongoing studies to test the effects of a device that radiates light into the ear—based on the theory that the light will pass through the skull and affect the brain directly. There is evidence that light introduced via the ear does in fact influence structures and chemicals within the brain. Whether this effect can be harnessed for therapeutic purposes remains to be seen. To date I have seen some encouraging pilot data but, as we know, placebo effects are powerful and the scientists will need to show, as with all clinical trials, that the ear light has specific therapeutic effects over and above placebo effects. Because such controlled study data are lacking to date, I would not recommend ear light at this time in favor of other forms of light therapy (such as the light box) whose safety and efficacy are well established. I am, however, interested in this new technology and open to changing my mind depending on the results of future studies.

Be sure to note that the effects of standard light therapy fixtures are quite different from those of lamps used in tanning salons (see question 43).

11. How far do I need to be from the box for light therapy to be effective?

The answer differs for different light boxes and different people. Usually, the distance at which the light is active will vary between 1 and 3 feet and should be specified by the manufacturer. According to simple laws of physics, the intensity of light exposure falls off sharply with the distance from a light source. Studies of light therapy have shown a relationship between the intensity of light exposure and the strength of the antidepressant effect. If you are to obtain the maximum therapeutic effect in the minimum amount of time, it is important to stay within the recommended distance from the light box.

12. What can I do while I am receiving light therapy?

You can do anything you like while receiving light therapy, provided your eyes are open, you are facing the box, and you are within the proper range. Some people use their light therapy sessions as an opportunity to catch up on chores, such as paperwork or returning business calls. But if this makes light therapy itself feel more like a chore, it may be better to use your light time for enjoyable activities like reading a novel or catching up with a friend on the phone. Some people like to relax in front of their light boxes, others to exercise. It is possible to set up a light box in front of an exercise machine (as in Figure 4), and some people have told me that the combination of light therapy and exercise is particularly energizing. Research bears out the benefits of combining these two forms of treatment.

One common concern people have is how to find time for daily light therapy in the midst of a busy schedule. Analyze your daily activities and determine when you will be seated in one place for a period of time each day. For light therapy to work best, it should be incorporated naturally into your current daily activities so it does not become an extra burden when you already feel overburdened. Almost everyone has at least some time during the day when they are sitting in one place. In fact, one common complaint about our nation's health is that we are *too* sedentary. If you can afford more than one light box, you can derive the benefits of light therapy by moving from one illuminated setting to another—say, from the kitchen table to the desk in your office—replicating the way we experience light in summer, when many of us feel at our best.

13. What is the best time of day to receive light therapy?

This question has been researched extensively, and the answer is that for most people light treatment is most effective if administered early in the morning. According to researchers Michael and Jiuan Su Terman, the earlier the better, especially if you are generally a morning person. The Termans have developed a formula that predicts what time of day light therapy will work best for you, based on how much of a morning versus evening person you are. (See *www.cet.org* for further information about this.) The trouble with getting light at the most effective time of day—as predicted by this formula—is that for many people the best times tend to be inconveniently early, thereby interfering with sleep. According to the Termans' studies, however, response rate to light therapy can double, from 40 to 80%, if treatments are shifted early enough, say from 8:00 A.M. to 6:00 A.M. In addition, using light therapy at an early hour of the day for several days tends to shift people's sleep schedules earlier, making it easier for them to fall asleep earlier in the evening and wake up earlier in the morning. This earlier schedule, however, doesn't work well for everyone.

Although most people can benefit from light therapy given at convenient times of the day, for some it may be critical to use light very early in the morning—like one of my patients, Hank. Unlike most people with SAD, who tend to become depressed in October or November, Hank would regularly become depressed toward the middle of August. Light therapy administered at conventional morning hours, such as 7:00 A.M.—even along with antidepressant medications—was unable to prevent Hank's inevitable slide into sluggishness and misery. Although mid-August is regarded as high summer, in fact at that time of year, dawn breaks about half an hour later than at the summer solstice. I wondered whether that missing half hour of light was triggering Hank's unusually early SAD symptoms. To test that theory, I asked Hank to start light therapy at 5:30 A.M., the time of dawn at the summer solstice in our part of the world. Both Hank and I were pleasantly surprised at his powerful response, which endured throughout the winter. Most people with SAD, however, do not need to wake up as early as Hank to benefit from light therapy.

One useful trick is to place a light box a few feet away from the bed and connect it to a timer that turns it on early in the morning. To avoid waking up with a jolt, it is best if the bright light follows an artificially simulated dawn, as described below (see question 36).

In practice, light therapy can be helpful when used at any time of day, including the evening hours. In addition, many benefit from using light therapy more than once a day, such as in the morning and the evening. If you are starting light therapy, try treatment first thing in the morning if your schedule permits. If you have been using light treatment in the morning with only partial benefit, try to shift sessions earlier in the morning. But if you still see no improvement, either switch to light therapy in the evening or add evening light therapy before concluding that you have obtained the maximum possible benefit.

14. For how long do I need to sit in front of the light box?

This varies from person to person and even within the same individual over the course of the year. Some people are exquisitely sensitive to light therapy, and 5 to 10 minutes per day are as much as they can take. I usually suggest such short treatments, at least initially, to those with a history of hypomania or mania, who may become unpleasantly wired by too much light therapy. Others may need to sit in front of their light boxes for hours. But most people end up using the box between 30 and 90 minutes (at 10,000 lux) per day, often divided into more than one light therapy session. This is either enough to have the desired effect or about as much time as they are willing to invest, in which case additional types of treatment may be needed.

If you are starting light therapy at the beginning of the winter season just as you are experiencing your first winter symptoms, start with about 20 minutes in the morning for the first week or so. If that reverses most of your symptoms without any untoward effects, stay with that duration until your body tells you that you need either more or less treatment. If you are still feeling the symptoms of SAD significantly after the first week, increase your treatment to about 45 minutes per day, either all in the morning or with no less than 30 minutes in the morning and the rest in the evening. Reevaluate your symptoms one week later and make adjustments again. You may find the chart at the end of this book of some help in evaluating your mood response (see Appendix A, p. 328).

If you experience side effects related to light therapy, such as irritability, anxiety, insomnia, headache, or eyestrain (a more complete list is provided in response to question 22), you may want to scale back the duration to, say, 10 or 15 minutes of therapy in the morning.

As the winter deepens, the degree of light deprivation increases and you will probably need to increase your duration of daily light therapy. It is important to be aware of this ahead of time so that you don't think that the treatment is no longer working for you. It is quite common, for example, to find that 20 minutes of light therapy per day is sufficient at the beginning of winter but that you need 90 minutes during January and February.

If you are already in the midst of your winter depression by the time you start light therapy, start with 20 minutes twice a day for a few days and then, after determining that there are no untoward effects, add an extra 10 minutes twice a day until you have reached a total daily exposure of 45 minutes twice a day. It is often worth allowing about 2 weeks at that dosage before deciding how effective the treatment is for you and whether any further steps need to be taken.

Remember, when the days begin to get longer and brighter in the spring, you will no longer need as much light therapy and will be able to taper off the duration of daily therapy accordingly. In fact, you may start to develop side effects in the spring, such as irritability and insomnia, indicating that you are receiving too much light therapy and need to cut back. After a while, you get good at recognizing whether you are receiving the right amount of light therapy per day: Too little and you begin to feel the symptoms of SAD again; too much and you feel wired, as though you have drunk too much coffee. Once you get the hang of it, you can add or subtract light so that you feel as good as possible. Even old light therapy veterans would do well to focus on how they feel each day and relate it to the amount of light they're getting. At times, I find myself reminding friends who have SAD to consider increasing their duration of light therapy, and if they see me slipping, they don't hesitate to return the favor.

15. Is it important to use full-spectrum light?

Full-spectrum light is a type of white light, fluorescent or incandescent, that mimics the colors of sunlight more closely than ordinary fluorescent lamps or incandescent lightbulbs. This type of light is often advertised as healthier than ordinary lighting, but there is no evidence in favor of these claims. Although many people prefer the color of full-spectrum fluorescent light, which appears a little bluer and a little less pink than ordinary fluorescents, they all probably work equally well.

Some full-spectrum lights emit more of a certain type of UV light than ordinary fluorescents, which may do more harm than good—because UV light is bad for the skin and the eyes. This risk factor is largely offset, however, by using a well-made light fixture with a proper UV filter on its diffusing screen. The bottom line as far as full-spectrum lamps are concerned is "Suit yourself." Feel free to use them if you prefer the color and are using a box with a UV filter, but don't feel obligated to go to any special lengths or pay any premium for this type of lamp.

16. Is it true that blue light is better than white light for treating SAD?

The reason that I am including this question is that several companies have marketed fixtures that emit blue light with claims or implications that they are better than standard white lights. To start with the bottom line: There is no evidence that blue light is better than conventional white light; some have raised concerns about the potential toxicity of blue light to the eyes; and finally, there are decades of experience about the safety and effectiveness of white light, which are lacking for blue light. Incidentally, the blue light in the fixtures I have seen comes from LEDs, which I have discussed in question 2.

> *Bottom line in the blue versus white light debate: White light is backed by decades of safe, effective use; there is no evidence that blue light is more effective; and some have voiced safety concerns about blue light.*

That said, let us consider some of the basic science behind these claims. All physiological effects mediated by the eyes depend on receptors in the retina, which contain specialized photopigments. Color vision, for example, depends on three different types of cone receptors that are especially sensitive at picking up certain wavelengths of light. Working together, these cones allow us to pick up different shades of color in the world around us. Another group of receptors, the rods, which use a different photopigment, are specialized for picking up light in dim surroundings. We depend on them for night vision.

In the past few decades scientists have discovered that light is capable of mediating many physical functions other than vision. It can suppress melatonin, shift circadian (daily) rhythms, make people more alert, and, yes, reverse the symptoms of depression in people with SAD. Researchers have attempted to tease out which receptors (or photopigments) are responsible for these nonvisual effects of light.

A novel photopigment called "melanopsin," which absorbs light most efficiently in the blue range, has been discovered in the retina. Several research groups, most notably that of George Brainard, Professor of Biochemistry and Molecular Pharmacology at Jefferson Medical College in Philadelphia, have explored which colors are most active in mediating nonvisual effects of light. Blue light has emerged as the leading candidate, possibly exerting its effects through the photopigment melanopsin. It is clearly possible—though not yet established—that blue light is most efficient in reversing the symptoms of SAD. But even if that turns out to be the case, that single finding should not overturn our years of experience with the safety and efficacy of white fluorescent light.

Incidentally, I and colleagues including Kathryn Roecklein, Assistant Professor in the Department of Psychology in the Uniformed Services University of the Health Sciences, have found that a variant of the gene that codes for melanopsin occurs more commonly in people with SAD than in the general population and may be responsible for symptoms in a small percentage of people with SAD.

17. Will light therapy still work if I take a break from it?

Yes. Short breaks in a light therapy session should not significantly decrease the overall benefit.

18. If one light box is good, would two be better?

Even though this question has never been studied systematically, based on my personal experience, I would say yes . . . sometimes. Some of my patients and I have at times boosted the effects of light therapy with extra light fixtures. But I don't recommend doing so without clinical supervision because all the side effects listed below (see question 22) could be aggravated by increasing the amount of light beyond ordinary recommended levels—just as the side effects of a medication can increase if you step up the dosage.

Teodor Postolache and others in my group at the NIMH found that individuals with SAD don't generally feel as well in the winter even with light therapy as they do in the summer. Postolache suggested that maybe the fragrances of summer improve mood and found that the smell of lemons actually boosts mood to a very small though significant degree in people with SAD. Another reason why summer may be more potent than a light box in reversing SAD symptoms, however, may relate to the surface area from which light emanates (the vast dome of the sky versus a light box). This second theory is consistent with the observation that two or three light boxes may be more effective than one.

19. Can I simply replace all the lamps in my house with full-spectrum lights?

This commonly asked question reveals a misunderstanding—namely, that the color tone of the light is important. As mentioned above, it not the color tone of the (basically white) light that matters, but the amount. So there is no reason to expect that replacing lightbulbs with those of a different hue will be more beneficial. So use only full-spectrum lights if you prefer them aesthetically to regular fluorescents.

20. Do I need to use light therapy every day? What happens if I skip a day or two? And when can I stop light therapy?

The result of skipping a day of light therapy will vary from person to person and will also depend on the season, the weather, and the amount of naturally occurring environmental light available. In the darkest depths of winter, most people with SAD need light on a daily or almost-daily basis. Some people manage quite well if they skip a *single* day of therapy, but after skipping therapy for 2 days or more, many feel some return of symptoms. One of my patients recognized this trend and asked not to participate in social activities that required him to skip light therapy for more than a single night during the winter.

Those who feel an immediate energizing effect of light therapy may be the first to miss therapy if they skip treatment for as little as a single day, whereas those who take longer to respond may also be able to do without light therapy for more days at a stretch. Just as low energy and difficulty getting out of bed in the morning are often the earliest symptoms of SAD, so they may be the first to return when treatment is discontinued.

When spring arrives, it may be possible to skip more days of light therapy without relapsing. Likewise, if you are out and about on a bright winter day, you may be able to do without treatment on that day. The principle here is simple. If you are getting enough light from some other source, it may be possible to skip formal light therapy without experiencing a relapse.

Another way to skip light therapy is to embrace one of the other treatment strategies outlined in subsequent chapters, such as embarking on a vigorous program of daily exercise or taking an antidepressant medication.

> *It is generally best not to skip more than 1 day of light therapy a week in order to feel well throughout the winter.*

21. Is there an advantage to starting light therapy early in the winter?

It is best to start light therapy as soon as the first symptoms of winter depression appear, before they progress to a full-blown picture of SAD. For some, this may be as early as August, while others may not begin to experience symptoms until January. Chapter 12, "A Step-by-Step Guide through the Revolving Year," deals with this question in greater detail.

22. What are the side effects of light therapy?

Light therapy is generally very well tolerated; side effects, when they occur, are usually mild. It is the rare individual who is unable to use light therapy altogether because of side effects. When they occur, the most common side effects of light therapy are:

- Headaches
- Eyestrain
- Irritability or anxiety
- Overactivity
- Insomnia
- Nausea

- Fatigue
- Dryness of the eyes
- Dryness of nasal passages and sinuses
- Sunburn-type reaction of the skin

Most of these side effects can be managed by decreasing the duration of treatment—for example, to 15 minutes per day—and then building it up gradually over a week or two to the more usual dosage. Alternatively, sit slightly farther away from the light source until symptoms subside. It is generally possible to move closer to the light box again after several days without experiencing a recurrence of these side effects.

Be sure, however, not to stare directly and close up at a light box (even one that has been approved for light therapy) for prolonged periods (say, more than 5 minutes at a time). There have been a small number of reports of eye sensitivity and severe headaches in people who have looked directly at the light in this way for extended periods of time.

Here are some additional points to bear in mind:

- *Irritability, anxiety, and overactivity.* People who become irritable during light therapy often compare those feelings to the way they feel during summer. Irritability, insomnia, increased energy, racing thoughts, and pressured speech are common symptoms of hypomania and mania. If you experience these symptoms, I suggest that you review the features of these conditions on pages 109–111. If the simple measures mentioned above to decrease light exposure fail to alleviate these side effects within a day or two, I suggest you consult your doctor without delay.

Although light therapy generally *decreases* the anxiety associated with SAD, in some people—usually the same ones who tend to become irritable or hypomanic—light therapy may *cause* anxiety, panic, and a feeling of overstimulation. One of my patients who developed these feelings on light therapy experienced stomach discomfort as part of her anxiety state, and at certain times of the year it was necessary to decrease the duration of light therapy—at times to as little as 5 minutes per day—to prevent this from happening. At other times of the year she was able to tolerate longer durations of treatment and, despite the anxiety, found light therapy to be very helpful overall.

• *Insomnia.* Insomnia is most apt to occur when the lights are used late at night. Some people complain that the lights make them feel too energized or "wired" to go to sleep. The best remedy is to shift treatment to an earlier time of day; even earlier in the evening may be fine.

• *Nausea.* According to Columbia University researchers Michael and Jiuan Su Terman, nausea is the one side effect that tends to go along with a favorable response to light therapy. As with some of the other side effects, the best remedy is to decrease the exposure until the nausea subsides and then gradually increase duration of treatment.

• *Fatigue.* Fatigue may occur after several days of light therapy, especially if the amount or timing of sleep has been changed to accommodate treatment. If feelings of fatigue persist, the best remedy is to try to get to bed earlier at night. Alternatively, it may be necessary to move treatment to a later hour in the morning, a less desirable choice as it may prove less effective at that time.

• *Dryness of eyes, nasal passages, or sinuses.* This problem may be due to the heat generated by the light box, which can dry out the surrounding air. In contact lens wearers, dry eyes may be more than just an irritant and may actually result in abrasions of the cornea. Artificial tears may help to overcome this problem, as may a humidifier placed in the vicinity of the light box, which may also relieve dryness of the nose and sinuses. Drinking hot beverages while undergoing treatment may also help. An added advantage to keeping the air humid is that humidity promotes a higher concentration of negative ions (charged particles) in the air, which may boost your mood (see pp. 188–190 for more information about this).

• *Reddening of the skin.* This problem, similar to a mild case of sunburn, may occur, especially in those with fair, sun-sensitive skin or in those taking certain medications that sensitize the skin to light. Such reddening is evidence that despite all attempts at removing ultraviolet rays, some of them are getting through the screen and reaching the skin. If this is a problem, consider using sunblock.

Suicide attempts or suicidal ideas have been reported, in very rare instances, within 2 weeks of starting light therapy. There is also one documented case of suicide after 5 days of light therapy. On the other hand, Raymond Lam, Professor of Psychiatry at the University of British Columbia, and his colleagues analyzed their clinic experience with

191 patients with SAD and found a significant *decrease* in suicidal tendencies in 45% following light treatment, with *only 3% showing worsening in these tendencies.* Since suicidal ideas and tendencies are part of mood disorders in general (and SAD is no exception here), it

If you experience any suicidal ideas before, during, or after light therapy, do yourself and everyone who cares about you a favor and report it to a health care professional without delay.

is reasonable to assume that they fluctuate to some degree as a result of fluctuations in the severity of the illness. It is therefore possible that the increases in suicidal ideas or tendencies seen in a small percentage of patients with SAD might have been unrelated to the light therapy. On the other hand, it is well known that increased activation in depressed people can sometimes bring out suicidal tendencies, as may also occur rarely following antidepressant treatment.

23. Is light therapy harmful to the eyes?

This question arises from time to time, especially in those who use light therapy year after year. The good news is that no problems of this type have arisen to my knowledge since light therapy first began to be used in the early 1980s, provided light therapy has been used as recommended and under proper supervision. The one isolated cautionary tale mentioned on page 129—the only one known to me where light therapy was clearly associated with an eye injury—occurred in someone who used a homemade light fixture in an unsupervised setting.

Two follow-up studies—one by Paul Schwartz and colleagues at the NIMH and the other by Chris Gorman and colleagues in Calgary, Canada—revealed no evidence of eye damage in, 59 and 71 patients, treated for an average duration of 9 years and 5 years, respectively. All these data were derived from people whose eye functioning was normal before treatment was initiated. They may not necessarily apply to people with abnormalities of visual functioning.

If you have any history of visual difficulties (apart from the need for ordinary corrective lenses), be sure to consult your eye doctor before undertaking light therapy. Certain retinal problems, such as macular degeneration and retinitis pigmentosa, can be made worse by exposure to bright light. These conditions may first appear as visual difficulties. Medications that sensitize the skin to sunlight (a property generally noted on the medication bottle or information sheet) may also sensitize the retina to bright light. Sometimes you can feel this effect. For example, some people on the herbal antidepressant St. John's wort have complained of eye pains during light therapy sessions. Sometimes, however, you may not be able to tell if there are toxic interactions between the light and the medications you are taking.

Although the concomitant use of photosensitizing medications has not generally been considered a reason to avoid light therapy, it does warrant extra caution. Be sure to draw your doctor's attention to the possible interaction and proceed more cautiously, for example, by increasing the duration of light therapy more gradually than is generally recommended or sitting a little farther away from the light box. It is possible that if you are taking a medication that sensitizes your tissues to light, you may derive benefit from lower doses of light than are generally needed.

The absence to date of any reported cases of eye problems related to light therapy is encouraging and is in keeping with our expectations, given the amount of light used in standard treatments. Even the highest-intensity (10,000-lux) light boxes give out no more light than you would receive if you looked at the horizon just after sunrise.

To minimize the possibility of any eye problems, it is important that manufacturers of light boxes screen out as much UV light as possible. Unfortunately manufacturers are not obliged to disclose how much UV light gets through the screens on their fixtures, and so far there are no Food and Drug Administration (FDA) guidelines for how much UV light transmission from therapeutic fixtures is acceptable. The good news is that a growing number of researchers and clinicians are treating ever-increasing numbers of patients for extended periods with no

> *There is no evidence to date that standard light therapy, when administered properly to individuals with normal visual functioning, is harmful to the eyes. But new fixtures using LEDs and blue light do not have the advantage of the years of safety data that exist for standard fluorescent light therapy devices.*

evidence of any eye problems so far. Of course, should you develop any eye-related symptoms while on light therapy, such as visual changes, irritation, or increased light sensitivity, check them out with your doctor promptly.

24. Should everyone have an eye examination before starting light therapy?

In practice, most clinicians and researchers do not routinely give eye examinations to people with normal visual functioning. If you have any problems with your eyes, however, check with your doctor before starting light therapy.

Before initiating light therapy eye exams should be given to anyone with a history of eye problems (over and above the need for corrective lenses) or to anyone in whom visual difficulties or eye-related symptoms develop during the course of ongoing light therapy. Absent these special circumstances, however, it is not standard practice to administer eye exams before initiating light therapy.

25. Is it safe for me to receive light therapy if I have sensitive skin?

As already mentioned, some UV rays get through the diffusing screen, and while these cause no problem for most people, they may lead to problems in those with sun-sensitive skin—including people with a history of skin cancers, those on medications that sensitize the skin to sunlight, and those with conditions, such as systemic lupus erythematosus, where there is enhanced sensitivity to sunlight.

For such light-sensitive individuals, I encourage the use of sunblock on the face, though even the most powerful of these creams may not screen out all the potentially damaging UV rays. If you have a history of skin cancer, check with your doctor before starting light therapy and have your skin monitored for possible recurrences at regular intervals. To put things in perspective, you will probably be exposed to far less UV light from your light box than from going outdoors. Even so, the UV rays coming from the light box may increase your chances of a recurrence of skin cancer. For this reason you and your physician should do a cost–benefit analysis of the potential benefits of light therapy to your mood versus the potential harm to your skin. Remember, many antidepressants sensitize the skin to environmental light and may also represent a risk factor for people with sensitive skin. On a reassuring note, I have come across several patients with a history of both lupus and SAD who have benefited from light therapy without suffering any skin problems.

26. How can I tell how likely I am to respond to light therapy?

Although it is not possible to predict exactly who is most likely to respond to treatment with bright light, the following factors predict a more favorable outcome:

- A history of mood improvement in the winter when you have been exposed to more light in a natural context, such as when you have traveled south or spent time in brighter indoor environments, or when you lived closer to the equator.
- Certain symptoms of winter depression, including fatigue, oversleeping, overeating, craving carbohydrates, weight gain, and social withdrawal.

In contrast, severely depressed people who lose sleep, eat less, and lose weight during their winter depressions tend to do less well with light therapy. But even if you *do* have these less favorable symptoms, light therapy is still worth a try if you have a clear-cut pattern of winter depressions, especially if your mood has been responsive to the amount of light in your environment.

One further predictor: if you feel a beneficial effect after 1 hour of light exposure, the chances are that you will continue to benefit over time.

27. What can I do if I dislike fluorescent lights?

Fluorescent lights make some people feel anxious, irritable, or wired. Such people are understandably concerned when fluorescent light fixtures are recommended as a treatment. In my experience, people with SAD rarely object to the quality of the light emanating from standard light-treatment fixtures; on the contrary, they generally find them relieving, soothing, or invigorating. Modern light fixtures contain special devices that minimize the irritating flicker that many associate with fluorescent lights.

People with seizure disorders, who have been told to avoid strobe lights, have wondered at times whether there is any reason to avoid light therapy. They will be relieved to learn that there is no evidence that standard light therapy fixtures pose any risk for seizures.

28. Is it safe to use light therapy while I am pregnant?

All evidence suggests that light therapy is safe for pregnant women, and I have known several pregnant women whose winter depressions have been treated successfully in this way and who have subsequently given birth to normal, healthy babies. In addition, Anna Wirz-Justice and colleagues conducted a controlled study of 23 depressed pregnant women and found that light therapy was superior to the control condition, without causing any particular problems for the mothers or their babies.

Besides having psychological problems, depressed people experience physical difficulties, such as sleep disruption, that might be bad for the developing baby. For the sake of both mother and baby, it makes sense to treat the physical and psychological symptoms of SAD, and it would seem far better to do so, if possible, without introducing any chemicals, such as antidepressant medications, into the system.

29. Can I use light therapy while nursing my baby?

Yes, but only if the infant's face is turned away from the light box. The eyes of an infant are far more sensitive than those of an adult and could potentially be harmed by the intense light emanating from a standard light fixture. So, if you decide to use light therapy while you are breastfeeding, be sure to shield the baby's face from the light.

30. Is it all right if older children are around the light box while I am being treated?

It is quite common for parents who are using light treatment to have children around, whether they are toddlers jumping on the parent's lap or older children with questions to ask or opinions to offer. Such casual light exposure should pose no problem. If the child has SAD, it might actually be beneficial to spend some time around the light box, and the companionship and identification with the parent that come from the shared experience can be very reassuring to a child or adolescent. I suggest, however, that you be protective of children under age 10, making sure they don't stare directly at the bright light.

31. Will the bright light be harmful to pets?

Many people have commented that their pets enjoy the lights. Cats in particular seem drawn to the light and are mesmerized by it. My favorite pet story involved a cat and a parakeet who was able to open his own cage. Ordinarily, when the cat encountered the bird, he would give chase and the parakeet would make a dash for his cage and slam the door shut behind himself. However, when the bright lights were turned on, the parakeet emerged from his cage and strutted in front of the light box, despite the dangerous proximity of the cat. The cat, for his part, appeared so entranced by the lights that he showed none of his usual interest in pursuing the parakeet. In summary, there is no reason to believe that any harm will come to your pet from sitting in front of your light box. Light can induce behavioral changes in animals just as it can in humans.

32. How can I handle other people's reactions to my light box?

Some people are embarrassed to have friends or colleagues see the light box. You may worry that they will speculate about what is wrong with you, make judgments about your competency or mental health, or ask embarrassing questions. It may also feel like an invasion of your privacy to have people speculating in this way.

Bringing a large box that emits intense light into an indoor environment is certain to have an impact on those around you. Those who use the light in work or home settings observe that some people are drawn to it and find it pleasant, while others may dislike it and find it irritating.

The concern that bringing a special light fixture into the workplace might label you in some way is understandable and may in some instances be well founded. Generally, you will have the best sense of how accepting the people at your work will be and whether it is advisable to use the lights in that setting or not. The reactions of colleagues might vary from one work setting to another. For example, colleagues and supervisors at a graphic design company or mental health center are likely to be more accepting of lights than officers at the CIA or the Pentagon, where it might be imprudent to bring the box in to work. Most people, however, have been pleasantly surprised at how accepting their colleagues are of the light box and the underlying condition that its presence implies. Perhaps that is because most people understand that seasons can affect behavior in animals, and many experience some seasonal changes themselves, albeit to a lesser degree. In fact, my patients have often told me how friends and colleagues tend to congregate around their light boxes on dreary days.

Questions about the lights are generally best handled in a matter-of-fact way, though one college student I know chose humor instead. When asked about the lights by his roommates, he replied that studies show that bright light maintains rats in a state of constant sexual arousal. That put an end to the questioning.

33. What should I do if light therapy doesn't start working within a week?

The 1-week mark is generally an excellent time to take stock of how your light therapy is working. If light therapy has not yet begun to work after 1 week, go through the following checklist:

- Make sure you are using the equipment correctly.
- Do you have the right sort of box? Is it large enough? (Remember, research studies have generally used light boxes about 1 foot high by 16 inches across.)
- Have you placed the box at eye level?

If the therapy is not helping at all after 1 week or is only partially helpful after 2 weeks, check in with your doctor or therapist (if someone is monitoring your treatment) or consider checking in with a professional if nobody is monitoring you. Above all, don't give up too soon, since significant improvements may take at least 2 weeks to occur.

- Are you sitting at the right distance from the fixture?
- Are you using the lights for long enough each day? Some people need at least 45 minutes in both the morning and the afternoon.
- It may be helpful to shift the treatment to a different time of day (usually earlier in the morning, but sometimes to the afternoon or evening).

34. What can I do if light therapy is helpful for a while but becomes less effective over time?

Although this problem may occur, it rarely means that light itself has lost its beneficial effects. A mood decline after an initial response may result from:

- A change in your life circumstances
- Decreased environmental light
- Inconsistent light treatment
- Loss of intensity of the fluorescent lamps

Consider each of these possibilities and ask yourself:

- "Has my life become more stressful in any way? For example, has anything changed at work or in my relationships?" If so, it is important to attend to the underlying stresses in your life so you can alleviate their effects on your mood.
- "Has it become darker outside?" Light treatment that is completely effective in November and December may become only partially effective in the darker days of January and February. In those months, the days are getting longer, but they are also often cloudier, so less light is available. To combat this climatic change, you may need to increase the amount of light or add some other type of treatment.
- "Have I been using the lights consistently, or have I slacked off, missed days, or cut my treatments short? Am I using the lights properly? For example, am I sitting at the right angle, so that my eyes are exposed to sufficient light?" Some people set the light to the side, thereby losing much of its benefit.
- "How old are the fluorescent lamps in my fixture?" After one

or two seasons of use, the amount of light given off by the lamps may decrease enough to diminish their effectiveness. If you are responding less well to treatment than you did previously and the lamps in your fixture are more than 2 years old, consider replacing them.

35. Do insurance companies cover light boxes?

Some people have successfully filed for insurance reimbursement for their light fixtures, but many people with SAD have had their claims denied, usually because light therapy is labeled "experimental" by the insurance company. The real reason, of course, is that insurance companies try to save money. The best strategy for obtaining reimbursement for your light fixture is to send the invoice for the light box to your insurance company along with a letter from your doctor. A sample of the sort of letter that I have sent for my patients is shown on page 152.

Two developments that would greatly enhance the extent to which light therapy units are reimbursed by insurance companies are (1) lobbying by patient advocacy groups and (2) approval of light fixtures as effective medical devices by the FDA. Unfortunately, patients with SAD have been less successful than those with other conditions at developing a support group. Such support groups typically have a variety of constructive agendas, which might include dealing with insurance companies. Insurance companies often look to the FDA to legitimize a medical device. This has not occurred with light boxes so far, largely because of the costs involved in getting such approval. Given that light therapy has been used since the early 1980s, however, and given the hundreds of scholarly articles documenting its benefits, resorting to this old excuse about the lack of FDA approval seems like a sorry attempt on the part of insurance companies to avoid paying for a legitimate medical expense. Nevertheless, it would be helpful if the FDA could weigh in constructively to help legitimize what has now become an old and time-honored technology.

36. Can I get my light therapy while I am asleep?

Surprisingly, you can get some benefit from light while you're sleeping. Researchers have found that simulating the light of a summer dawn helps those with SAD wake up in the morning and feel better during

Sample Letter for Insurance Reimbursement

To Whom It May Concern:

This is to certify that Ms. Jane Smith has been a patient of mine since _____. I have treated her for recurrent major depressions (DSM-IV-TR 296.3), with a seasonal pattern. This condition, also known as seasonal affective disorder (SAD), has been shown in many studies in the United States and elsewhere in the world to respond to treatment with bright environmental light (light therapy). Light therapy is no longer considered experimental but is a mainstream type of psychiatric treatment, as evidenced by its inclusion in the authoritative *Treatments of Psychiatric Disorders, Third Edition,* a publication of American Psychiatric Publishing.[1] The effectiveness of light therapy was further confirmed in a 2005 meta-analysis published in the prestigious *American Journal of Psychiatry.*[2] To administer light therapy adequately, a light box, such as the one named in the attached invoice, is required.

Although a light box is an expensive piece of equipment, the experience of clinicians who have used it for many patients indicates that it saves a great deal of money over time by reducing the number of doctors' visits and the costs of medications and laboratory investigations of persistent symptoms, as well as the indirect costs of lost productivity. I maintain that in Ms. Smith's case, the use of such a light fixture should be regarded not only as a medical necessity, to be used in preference to, or in addition to, other forms of treatment, but also as a means of reducing her overall medical costs.

---

[1]Oren, D. A., & Rosenthal, N. E. (2001). Light therapy. In G. O. Gabbard (Ed.), *Treatments of psychiatric disorders* (3rd ed., Vol. 2, pp. 1295–1306). Washington, DC: American Psychiatric Publishing.

[2]Golden, R. N., Gaynes, B. N., Ekstrom, R. D., Hamer, R. M., Jacobsen, F. M., Suppes, T., et al. (2005). The efficacy of light therapy in the treatment of mood disorders: A review and meta-analysis of the evidence. *American Journal of Psychiatry, 162*(4), 656–662.

the day. This should make sense to many people (and not only those with SAD) who are aware that on a sunny day they wake up in the morning and jump out of bed even before they realize what type of day it is outside. In contrast, on a dreary, cloudy day it may be difficult to pull yourself out from under the covers even before looking out of the window and identifying the reason for the problem—a bank of cumulus clouds blocking the sunlight. Presumably, in the final hours of sleep, the eyes register the quality of ambient light and send signals to the brain that help you decide whether to jump out of bed or linger under the covers.

I recommend that people with SAD obtain a device called a dawn simulator, which can be attached to a bedside lamp (or houses its own light source) and turns on gradually in the early morning before the intended wake-up time. Researchers Michael and Jiuan Su Terman at Columbia Psychiatric Institute originally suggested the use of such dawn simulators, which were later tested extensively by David Avery and colleagues at the University of Washington in Seattle.

One such dawn simulator, the SunUp, shown in Figure 5, is a small electronic gadget that fits into the palm of one's hand and can be plugged into an ordinary bedside lamp. Advantages of the SunUp are (1) its compact size, which is perfect for travelers—I don't leave home without it when traveling in the winter; (2) the fact that you can plug it into any incandescent lamp (though not fluorescent lamps); (3) its flexible programming capacity, which enables the user to regulate the duration of the artificial dawn—the interval between complete darkness and the maximum intensity of the light source; and (4) substantial research demonstrating its effectiveness in reversing the symptoms of SAD.

I recommend attaching the dawn simulator to a lamp containing a lightbulb of no more than a 60- to 100-watt intensity and programming it to create an artificial dawn lasting between 30 and 60

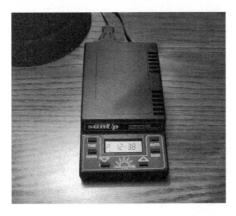

FIGURE 5. The SunUp dawn simulator.

minutes. Your eyes are very sensitive to light in the early-morning hours, and a bedside lamp that is too bright may disrupt sleep and cause irritability and overactivation. If this occurs after you have started to use a dawn simulator, decrease the intensity of the light source, increase the distance of the lamp from your pillow, or shorten the duration of the artificial dawn.

If incandescent lights are phased out completely because of their energy inefficiency, dawn simulators will either have to be modified to work with compact fluorescents (which is not currently the case) or they will need to use other light sources, such as halogen lamps or LEDs. This particular use for LEDs seems quite appropriate—very different from using them for light therapy as the user will not need to stare directly at the LEDs.

Two other popular dawn simulators are the Rise and Shine Light and the SunRise Clock, which contain an alarm clock and light source in a single device (see Figures 6a and 6b). A handy new travel version of the SunRise Clock is also available and is certainly worth considering (Figure 6c).

It is curious that dawn simulation works while users are asleep with their eyes shut, especially given the low intensity of the light source, as compared with a light box. The beneficial effects of the dawn simulator are best explained by the heightened sensitivity of the eyes in the predawn hours.

In choosing a dawn simulator, consider the pros and cons of having the light source embedded within the device (convenience, appeal-

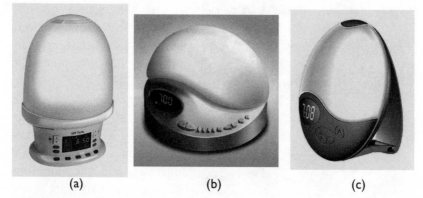

(a)   (b)   (c)

FIGURE 6. (a) **The Rise and Shine Light by Verilux.** (b) **The SunRise Clock by BioBrite.** (c) **The travel version of the SunRise clock.**

ing design, all-in-one convenience) versus a device that attaches to your bedside lamp (you choose the light source, which is better positioned for shining down on your face, as occurs with a natural dawn). New devices appear on the market with such frequency that any comprehensive list I might try to construct is soon likely to become obsolete.

Interestingly, the very first alarm clock ever invented incorporated both sound and light in its mechanism. It was the first profitable invention of Jean Eugene Robert-Houdin (1805–1871), who created a gadget containing a bell that would ring to wake the sleeper and a lighted candle that came out of a box.

37. If I have to choose one light treatment device, should I go with the light box or the dawn simulator?

I would hate to have to choose, because light boxes and dawn simulators make a great combination. Of the two, however, studies suggest that the light box is more potent. But the two devices work well together, the dawn simulator helping you wake up and get your day going while the light box provides extra light to help reverse the symptoms of SAD. Remember, if you cannot afford a specialized dawn simulating device, you can still create an artificial dawn—albeit a rather abrupt one—by plugging your bedside lamp into an ordinary timer, which costs only a few dollars. Evidence suggests that this less expensive solution may work perfectly well.

38. What about creating an artificial dusk? Is there any advantage to that?

All the dawn simulating devices described here permit the user to generate an artificial dusk by turning the light source off gradually until the bedroom is completely dark. Although there is no evidence that the dusk feature confers any benefit in the treatment of SAD, it can be very helpful for people with insomnia or disturbances of their daily rhythms. Some parents have also observed that it has been helpful for children who are afraid to go to sleep in a darkened room but have difficulty falling asleep with the light on. In some cases, an artificial dusk has resolved this difficulty.

One useful feature of the dawn simulator is that it permits a person to gradually increase or decrease the intensity of the bedside lamp without disrupting the programming of dawn or dusk. This feature is helpful at night if one person in a couple comes to bed later than the other. The dawn simulator allows you to turn the bedside lamp on very gradually at night so as not to disturb your partner. It also allows you to turn the light off gradually when you want to go to sleep. Gradually decreasing the intensity of the light in the bedroom helps slow down your thoughts and ease the transition between the day's activities and the night's rest.

39. How about receiving light therapy by means of a head-mounted light device?

Warning: Even though the light visor permits you to move around while receiving light therapy, some activities—such as driving, operating machinery, and walking up or down stairs or in hazardous areas—are not recommended during therapy with this device.

Although head-mounted devices do not have the same track record in controlled studies as light boxes or dawn simulators, some people have found them helpful and have enjoyed their portability (see Figure 7). They have the advantage of small size and low weight, which make them useful for travelers. Once again, new models frequently appear on the market, so I advise you to shop carefully not only for prices but also to make sure that light sources don't have "hot spots"—points of intense brightness—and are properly screened for UV light.

40. Could I get my light therapy by making a whole room in my house bright enough?

The answer is yes, but it would take some doing. This is how light therapy is often administered in Sweden, either in a clinic setting or in a "light

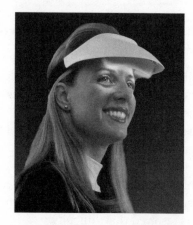

FIGURE 7. The light visor by BioBrite.

café," where people come for their regular light fix during the dark winter days. I had the good fortune of visiting one such room at St. Gjöran's Hospital in Stockholm, a center for light therapy research in Sweden. All the lighting in the room was indirect—emanating from recessed fluorescent tubes reflected off the white ceiling and walls. To increase the amount of reflected light, the overstuffed chairs and sofas were all draped with white sheeting and all visitors were given white hospital clothes to cover their street clothes.

The atmosphere in the room was otherworldly. It was October when I visited Stockholm, and there was a definite wintry feeling in the air. The sun, slung low on the horizon, offered a chilly welcome, and despite the warm and friendly reception from friends and colleagues, I could feel the juice ebbing out of me. That changed after 30 minutes in the light room. The immediate effect was extremely pleasant, both calming and energizing. Sitting there, I felt my energy return to me just in time to be appropriately animated for my presentation.

If you want to replicate this effect in a room in your house, you might try to incorporate the same elements used by the Swedes, namely:

- Indirect lighting—fluorescents are best to minimize heat
- White walls
- Light carpeting and furniture
- White spa-type robes for everyone in the room

A bright and cheerful room, even if it falls far short of the Swedish ideal, can be very therapeutic. Consider making one room in your house your "light room."

One of my patients with SAD, a physician himself, spent a lot of time in his kitchen and decided that would be the best room to modify. He went to the trouble of actually installing lights in the cabinetry—a degree of remodeling that should not be necessary.

OTHER WAYS TO BOOST INDOOR LIGHT LEVELS

- Wash windows, trim hedges around them, and remove low-lying branches near the house.

- Skylights. If you don't want to go to all that trouble, consider installing a SunPipe—a shiny aluminum tube that extends from the outside of the roof to just below the ceiling.

- Find ways to use bright colors and surfaces to good effect. Replace dark wood paneling with walls covered in light-colored paint or wallpaper. Splashes of yellow and orange on curtains and cushions also seem to work well, as do white or off-white carpeting and furnishings.

- Before buying a new home, pay attention to the size of the windows and the directions that the rooms face. If you purchase a house during spring or summer, think of how it will look in the winter. One of my patients bought a house in a pine forest during the summer, not realizing that during the winter the sun would be closer to the horizon and the evergreens would cast their shadows across the house. That caused him to go into one of his worst winter depressions ever.

41. If there is more light outdoors on a winter's day than I get from my light box, why not just go for a walk instead of doing light therapy?

It is true that if you stare at the sky (never directly at the sun!) on a bright winter day, you will be exposed to more light than you get from a light box. But the same would not apply for a cloudy day, of which there may be many during the course of a winter, depending on where you live. In other words, winter days are unreliable. In addition, they can be cold and unpleasant, and when you are depressed, you may be disinclined to walk outdoors regularly. A light box in a cozy room is generally a more practical proposition. Even if there is a lot of light coming off the sky, you may not benefit much from it as most people do not gaze upward when they walk. They are more likely to focus on the landscape, and the amount of light coming off the ground and winter vegetation is often minimal and certainly variable. On the other hand, when the ground is covered with snow, there may be more than enough light around. (You may even need to wear sunglasses!)

In one study, Anna Wirz-Justice and colleagues in Basel, Switzerland, found that walking outdoors for 30 minutes each morning was very therapeutic for their patients with SAD. But the winter weather where you are may not be as conducive to good spirits as in Switzerland, and you may find it difficult to muster up the same degree of discipline as Wirz-Justice's Swiss patients. While walking outdoors is an excellent way to supplement your light therapy program, it is probably impractical for most people to rely on this alone.

Surprisingly, even in sunny places it may be important to go outdoors during the day. According to one Hawaiian psychiatrist I interviewed, his patients with SAD develop symptoms because they don't venture out into the sunlight. He has found that simply encouraging them to do so can ensure they get sufficient light to control their depressive symptoms.

42. Is it possible to combine light therapy with antidepressant medications?

It is commonplace to use these different types of treatment together. Light therapy can be used in conjunction with any antidepressant, which often allows lower dosages of antidepressants to be used, resulting in fewer undesirable side effects.

43. Will it help to go to a tanning salon?

Although research shows that light therapy fixtures work via the eyes and not the skin, some people with SAD report immediate mood improvement following visits to tanning salons. A scientific study by Steven R. Feldman and colleagues at Wake Forest University Baptist Medical Center in Winston-Salem, North Carolina, lends credence to patients' reports. The researchers placed the volunteers in tanning beds with and without ultraviolet filters (without telling them which was which) on 2 successive days. On the third day subjects were allowed to choose which tanning bed they wanted to use, and 11 out of 12 chose the bed with the UV rays.

Other research shows that UV light can cause certain skin cells to release the substance beta-endorphin, an opiate-like substance that may account for UV light's euphoriant effect. Although UV light on the skin may improve mood, I recommend against such tanning sessions because of the known potential for these rays to cause skin cancers, including potentially deadly melanomas.

44. How does light therapy stack up against antidepressant medications?

In two studies researchers compared light therapy to Prozac. Essentially, both found the two treatments to be roughly equivalent, though light therapy kicked in quicker. These results are good news for people with SAD, who have a choice of effective treatments for their condition. The use of medications for SAD is covered in greater detail in Chapter 10. Remember, light therapy and medications often work very well together, boosting each other's effects or allowing a person to feel well with a lower dosage of each.

Creating a Light Therapy Program That Works for You

As you can see, there are many different ways of boosting your environmental light. Most people prefer combining strategies in a way that maximizes the overall amount of daily light exposure through the season of risk. But remember, SAD symptoms can appear at unexpected times if the weather becomes cloudy. So be ready to use light therapy out of season if necessary. Ideally, a comprehensive light therapy program involves moving seamlessly from one light-enhanced environment to another at different times of day. Perhaps the best example I can offer is my own light treatment program. As you will see, I also use other, nonmedical types of treatment, which I will share with you in later chapters.

My Personal Winter Routine

When people ask me whether I suffer from SAD myself, I know the answer is yes, though it has been years since I have experienced the symptoms of the condition in a sustained way to any significant degree. The reason for this is that for many years I have taken a series of measures to keep these symptoms at bay. I suspect that without all these preventive actions I might not do too well, especially since my work as a clinician and SAD researcher has often meant that winter is my busiest and most stressful season.

My typical winter day begins at 6:00 A.M., when my dawn simulator is set to turn on my bedside lamp. Although I am still asleep at that time, I can imagine the lampshade gradually becoming brighter as the light enters the pupils of my eyes through my closed eyelids. At 7:00 A.M. my first alarm clock begins to ring, and the process of turning it off ensures that my head comes out from under the covers and my eyelids open wide enough to let in a fair amount of light. By this time, my bedside lamp has reached its maximum intensity, and all of a sudden a light box, 3 or 4 feet from my head, set on a timer, goes on and my eyes are exposed to about 2,500 lux of light. Believe it or not, I continue to doze as I stir, aware that the end of the night is rapidly approaching. It takes the second alarm clock, set for 7:30 A.M., to bring that message finally home to me, and I am able to get out of bed fairly easily. This stands in sharp contrast to those days when, for whatever reason, the lights do not come on, and I feel that I have to drag myself out of a coma to get up.

I meditate for 20 minutes (see Chapter 11 for more details), then check my e-mail at a computer flanked by two light boxes. I have found that this setup allows me to see the computer screen clearly while receiving light from both sides.

I walk outdoors in the morning in all sorts of weather and reserve an elliptical trainer only for days when there is ice on the ground. I often walk with a friend and find that unless I make a commitment to meet someone at a set time, the temptation to play hooky is very great. Working out in the morning seems to energize me for the rest of the day.

After my workout it's time for breakfast in a sunroom while I read the paper in front of a light box before starting my work. I also have a light box in my office, which my patients often ask me to turn on during sessions.

After people have been using light therapy for some time, they rarely need to calculate exactly how much light exposure they have had on a given day and how much more they need. It becomes instinctive. When they feel sluggish and lethargic, they can tell that they need more light. On the other hand, when they have had too much light, they typically feel a sort of edginess, as though they have had too much coffee. It is important to develop this ability so that you can gauge your own light requirements, since they vary over the course of the winter and no single regimen will work all the time. I recommend that you develop the skill of focusing your attention inward to evaluate whether you have had the right amount of light and to adjust your light exposure schedule accordingly.

Many people who have used the type of light treatment regimen I outline above—supplemented by planned winter retreats to sunny places—have told me that it is sufficient to keep them on an even keel through the winter. In fact, some people with SAD have told me that they now look forward to winter as a season with its own pleasures and rewards (see Chapter 17 for more information).

I have my eyes checked regularly (though no more frequently than I would if I didn't have SAD), and I am pleased that the ophthalmologist has found no problems even though I have used light therapy since the early 1980s.

Since the details of life vary from person to person, my program may not be right for you. I recommend that you use creativity in developing a light therapy program that works for you. It may take a while to learn how to make your life easier during the difficult winter months— but the effort is well worth the trouble.

Here's an example of someone who has successfully developed her own light therapy program, courtesy of one reader who wrote me from Albuquerque, New Mexico:

> I would like to see you discuss how important it is to work with the lights in order to fine-tune them to one's own needs (which can be very unique). Thanks to light therapy, in 1993 I had my first depression-free winter in ten years. But—the light box did not work by itself!! It did work in the early fall, when the sun was still coming up pretty early. But when the mornings were dark, the box ceased working—no matter how long I used it or at what time. I carefully read all the various books—to no avail.
>
> Almost hopeless, I asked myself what was wrong and realized that what I craved was to be submerged in light—like I was sitting on a beach. Sitting in relative darkness, with regular home lighting, focusing on a single strong light source (the light box) didn't feel "right" to me. I followed my instincts, set up my light box in my bedroom, along with all my old homemade light boxes—a total of eight four-foot-long fluorescents,

which had worked moderately well in past winters (if I used them for four hours a day!). I submerged myself in light in the mornings—and that's what turned the switch on again. And it stayed on consistently through the winter. How do I know I have gotten my dose? My hands tingle! It's like the circuit is connected.

Here are this person's thoughts about doctors who have been dismissive of her symptoms or have given her casual advice that has not gone far enough in addressing the seriousness of her winter problems:

Soon I hope the doctors in this area will stop saying, "You can't have SAD in Albuquerque—it's sunny here." Don't they read? . . . Beware of doctors who claim that "going out for an hour a day," adding more lightbulbs in home fixtures, etc., is all you need. This is what I was told by various psychiatrists—of course, it didn't work, and I discovered what I need to do only through my own reading and my depression support group.

This reader has discovered the critical importance of using her own inventiveness, taking some responsibility for her own treatment, customizing it to her needs, and not relying entirely on her doctors. I encourage you to do the same, but if you stray from regular treatment guidelines, be sure to involve your physician.

Other Therapeutic Applications of Light Therapy

One of the most exciting recent developments in the field of light therapy is its value for conditions other than SAD or the milder winter blues. In thinking about the benefits of bright light exposure, it is worth considering two sets of conditions: (1) disturbances of circadian (daily) rhythms and (2) other psychiatric conditions. Although the two are addressed separately below, keep in mind that they may overlap. For example, circadian disturbances may be at the core of some psychiatric conditions. For more information than what follows, see the Further Reading section in Part IV (Resources).

Disturbances of Circadian Rhythms

There are several circumstances in which the body's clock can be out of sync with the outside world and its rhythm of day and night. In some cases, this maladjustment may be temporary, such as when people fly across several time zones and develop jet lag or when they work changing shifts. In other cases, however, it may be a permanent state resulting from some internal abnormality of the body clock. The second category includes people who are extreme "night owls," who cannot fall asleep until very late at night and cannot wake up easily at conventional hours—a condition known as "delayed sleep phase syndrome" (DSPS). On the other end of the sleep–wake spectrum are those with "advanced sleep phase syndrome" (ASPS), who tend to fall asleep early in the evening and wake up early in the morning. Many elderly people fall into this category.

All the circadian rhythm disturbances mentioned have two things in common. First, they all result in discomfort and difficulties if the people involved are expected to adhere to a schedule that is at odds with their body clock and are not free to sleep and wake when they choose. Second, they can all be helped by appropriate adjustments in exposure to light and dark.

Understanding how exposure to light and dark can affect the timing of the body's clock requires some appreciation of what is known as the phase response curve (or PRC). All creatures studied to date, from single-celled organisms to human beings, show a PRC to light. This curve describes the relationship between the time of an animal's 24-hour day when it is exposed to light and the resulting effect on its circadian rhythm on subsequent days. For example, light exposure late at night tends to push these rhythms later on the following days. On the other hand, light exposure in the early hours of the morning, say at 6:00 A.M., tends to push these rhythms earlier on the following days. Staying in the dark has just the opposite effects on daily rhythms.

Delayed and Advanced Sleep Phase Disorder

My colleagues and I at the NIMH found that bright light exposure in the morning, together with avoidance of bright light in the evening, helps extreme "night owls" (those with delayed sleep phase syndrome, or DSPS) to readjust their sleep–wake schedules to more conventional hours. In other words, they can get to sleep and wake up more easily at "normal" times.

For people with late-night jobs, such as actors or bartenders, a delayed sleep pattern may fit in well with their lifestyle. But when extreme "night owls" choose—or are required—to live on a 9:00 to 5:00 schedule, they are likely to have problems. For example, businessmen, stockbrokers, and accountants may be unable to succeed at their jobs because they can't get in to work on time and therefore miss out on the crucial early-morning hours. DSPS is not uncommon among adolescents and young adults, who may struggle—at times unsuccessfully—to get to their early morning classes and have school difficulties as a consequence. Many of these teenagers find that even when they can get their bodies into class, they would rather be in bed and are unable to concentrate during the morning hours. For those who cannot easily adapt their lives to their sleep schedules, the good news is that it is possible to readjust their sleep–wake schedules to more conventional times.

Light therapy is being used increasingly to help people treat insomnia—even those without clear-cut delayed or advanced sleep phase disorder. In general, keeping lighting levels low in the evening and bright in the morning helps people get to sleep and wake up earlier. Also, amplifying the natural rhythms of day and night can help consolidate sleep in some people with insomnia.

Advanced sleep phase syndrome (ASPS), a condition found most frequently among the elderly, responds to a pattern of light exposure opposite to that required for treating DSPS. These people should be exposed to bright light in the evening and stay in relatively dim light in the early morning.

Jet Lag

Jet lag is a condition in which the rhythms of the body clock are temporarily out of sync with those of the external world as a result of traveling across time zones. The condition can persist for 10 days or even longer, depending on the number of time zones crossed and a person's ability to shift circadian rhythms. In its milder forms, jet lag can be a nuisance, causing people to wake up when they want to sleep and doze off when they should be awake. Appropriately timed exposures to bright light and darkness can greatly diminish the length of time necessary to shift a person's rhythms into sync with local time. To find out when it is best to use light or stay in the dark, depending on how many time zones you have traveled and in what direction, see the Resources (Part IV), where I refer you to a book that my colleagues and I wrote on this specific topic.

Nowadays, however, taking melatonin tablets is often a more convenient alternative. One simple formula is to take 3 milligrams of melatonin (an over-the-counter preparation) at about 9:00 P.M. on the plane (assuming you are leaving at night) and then at bedtime in the new location for as long as necessary until you have established circadian rhythms appropriate to your new location.

Shift Work

Just as those suffering from jet lag experience distress as a result of being fatigued when they are supposed to be alert and suffer sleep difficulties, so do shift workers, who can be considered to be chronically "jet-lagged" as a result of their shifting work schedules and disruption of their sleep times. The circadian problems of shift workers can induce not only discomfort—or even physical illness—in the worker, but also sleepiness on the job—and errors in judgment can result in serious industrial accidents. The nuclear accidents at Chernobyl and Three Mile Island both occurred in the early hours of the morning, and researchers have speculated that worker error might have resulted from fatigue and circadian disruption.

Just as properly timed exposure to bright light and dark can be used to help those suffering from jet lag, they can also be used to help night shift workers, according to Charmane Eastman, Professor of Behavioral Sciences at Rush University Medical Center in Chicago. Eastman and her colleagues have developed protocols for using bright light and dark at specific times to help night shift workers. She warns against simple remedies, such as "Try 30 minutes of bright light each morning," pointing out that light, if administered at the wrong time, can sometimes delay adjustment to the new shift. Because of the complexity of getting the timing of light and dark exactly right, I recommend shift workers look up Eastman's work on this topic.

Other Psychiatric Disorders

Several psychiatric disorders get worse in the winter. These include mood disorders with a seasonal component, eating disorders (both bulimia and anorexia), and premenstrual disorder. Given their seasonality, these conditions have been considered logical candidates for light therapy—often with good effects.

Bulimia

Controlled studies conducted by Raymond Lam and other researchers have shown that light therapy is superior to a control treatment for bulimia. Here is a description of one of his patients:

PHYLLIS: "I JUST CAN'T STOP BINGEING"

Phyllis, a travel agent, was 24 when she appealed to Dr. Lam during the winter for help with bulimia. "I lose control of myself," she confessed to him. "I can eat two boxes of crackers or a dozen cookies within an hour. Then I make myself vomit. Afterwards, I feel awful—guilty and angry at myself. I am preoccupied with my weight and unhappy with the shape of my body—5 feet 4 inches and 130 pounds, 10 of which I gained last winter." Phyllis described how in the past she had downed laxatives and exercised until she was ready to drop in an attempt to get to her "ideal" weight. Besides her bulimia, Phyllis had been quite depressed in the months before visiting Dr. Lam.

Dr. Lam treated Phyllis with light therapy—10,000 lux for 30 minutes per day in the early morning. After 2 weeks, her mood brightened and her energy and concentration improved. So did the bingeing, which settled down to its much

Important Tip: People with bulimia may respond to light therapy even if their symptoms are not seasonal, but those whose binges get worse in the winter may be the most promising candidates.

lower summer pattern after a month of treatment. She then entered a cognitive-behavioral group psychotherapy program, which helped her stop bingeing entirely. She continued to use light treatment, reporting cheerfully that "I've gained back the lost winter months."

Premenstrual Syndrome

When Barbara Parry worked at the NIMH, she realized that many women with SAD also have PMS, which often gets worse in winter. That led Parry to wonder whether light therapy might benefit people with PMS—and, after several controlled studies, she found that it does! Now a professor of psychiatry at the University of California in San Diego, Parry offered the following description of one of her patients.

Joan: A Teacher with PMS

Joan was a 33-three-year-old sixth-grade schoolteacher when she entered Dr. Parry's program. Her premenstrual symptoms had begun some 5 years earlier, after the birth of her first child. Initially these symptoms lasted only 2 to 3 days, but they worsened over time to occupy about 2 weeks of every menstrual cycle, from shortly after ovulation until 2 or 3 days after the start of her menstrual period. During these days a sense of "doom and gloom" settled over her. She felt inadequate as a wife, mother, teacher, and woman. All she wanted to do was to "hibernate"—to sit on the sofa and eat "bon-bons." She slept poorly, woke frequently during the night, and felt tired the following day. She avoided social engagements, was irritable with the kids and her husband, had no motivation, and easily broke down in tears. She wanted to "get away from it all" and even thought of admitting herself to a hospital.

Joan entered Dr. Parry's light treatment study because she didn't want to take drugs and get "all those bothersome side effects." She had tried treating her symptoms with vitamin B_6, which is commonly used for PMS, without success. But with light therapy, the outcome was completely different. She responded within 3 to 4 days of treatment (10,000 lux for 30 minutes), preferring treatment sessions in the evening rather than the morning, when it made her feel as though she had drunk too many cups of coffee. The evening light also allowed her to stay up later and spend more quality time with her husband. After the study she continued to use lights on a monthly basis, starting a week before her period was due. Light therapy remained just as effective over time as it had been at the beginning. When she was asked to stop the light therapy for 1 month for research purposes, her symptoms returned right away and in full force—a clear indication of how important her monthly treatments are.

Non-SAD Depression

One of the most exciting potential uses for light therapy is for non-SAD depression. You may recall my colleague with summer SAD who treated her symptoms effectively by going out into the sun in the early morning during the summer. Or the successful study of pregnant women with depression by Anna Wirz-Justice and colleagues. These are just a few examples showing a profound benefit of light therapy for nonseasonal depression.

In an exciting 2011 study, Risaert Lieverse, currently a psychiatrist and researcher in the School of Mental Health and Neuroscience at Maastricht University in the Netherlands, spearheaded a controlled study of bright light (7,500 lux for 60 minutes early in the morning) in 89 older people (60 years or more) with depression. They found that bright light was not only superior to the control treatment as an antidepressant but also reduced levels of the stress hormone cortisol in both urine and saliva. The latter finding is especially interesting as elevated levels of cortisol in blood, saliva, and urine are a hallmark of people with nonseasonal depression, where they have been interpreted as evidence of increased stress in these people. The reduction of cortisol in depressed people following light therapy further corroborates its authentic beneficial effects in this group. Curiously, elevated cortisol levels have never been described in people with SAD even though they may be just as depressed as—or more depressed than—people with nonseasonal depression.

An extraordinary use of light therapy for people with nonseasonal depression is as one of the three elements of triple chronotherapy—the other two elements being wake therapy (also known as sleep deprivation) and phase advance of sleep (also known as asking people to go to sleep and wake up earlier than normal). These last two interventions are known to have antidepressant effects in their own right. By combining all three elements together, researchers have found a highly potent and, more important, an enduring antidepressant effect of this combination of nondrug therapies. In fact, so powerful is this combination that in Milan, Italy, where much of this research has been done by Francesco Benedetti, head of research at the Division of Neuroscience at San Raffaele, triple chronotherapy is often used as an alternative to shock therapy in treating the most severely depressed patients. For more details as to exactly what triple chronotherapy involves, I refer you once again to the Resources at the back. At this point, however, I simply want to point out that it is just one more use for what has become an extraordinarily versatile form of treatment—light therapy.

Let me conclude this chapter with Goethe's famous words, quoted above—*"Mehr licht"*—more light. More light is what people with SAD need, but there is much more to light therapy that we have yet to discover. Once the new kid on the block, light therapy has now come of age. I look forward to watching its continued development in the years to come.

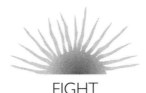

EIGHT

Beyond Light Therapy

OTHER WAYS TO HELP YOURSELF

Live in rooms full of light
Avoid heavy food
Be moderate in the drinking of wine
Take massage, baths, exercise, and gymnastics
Fight insomnia with gentle rocking or the sound of running
    water
Change surroundings and take long journeys
Strictly avoid frightening ideas
Indulge in cheerful conversation and amusements
Listen to music
      —A. CORNELIUS CELSUS, physician, first century A.D.

> ▶ Are you still left with some symptoms after starting light therapy?
>
> ▶ Are you interested in exploring other self-help strategies that might help before seeing a professional for psychotherapy or antidepressant medications?
>
> In most light therapy studies, more than one-third of patients fail to respond completely to active light therapy. Luckily, there are many other ways for people with SAD to help themselves overcome winter depression—or, indeed, depression at any time of

the year. In this chapter I will discuss other things that you can do yourself to make winter a more cheerful season. I've devoted an entire chapter (Chapter 11) to meditation, which you may find quite helpful. If your problems are severe, or you feel you might benefit from professional help, you'll find information on psychotherapy and medications in Chapters 9 and 10.

Understanding SAD: The First Step

One of the most useful things about having diagnosed SAD is that it provides you with a new way of understanding your difficulties. Notwithstanding the many years since we first described SAD, the condition remains underdiagnosed and undertreated. Large-scale studies conducted in the early 2000s found that fewer than 50% of patients with SAD had been treated for their condition, even though they had suffered through an average of 13 winter depressions. Diagnosis is the key to proper treatment. In addition, it is important to appreciate just how much the symptoms of SAD can rob you of your ability to function and enjoy yourself during the precious winter months.

It is one thing to understand intellectually that you have SAD, but another to acknowledge the degree to which it is interfering with your capacity to enjoy yourself or to be productive. I have seen many people suffer needlessly winter after winter simply because they have had trouble accepting the severity of their condition and its impact on their lives. One woman, for example, after being diagnosed with SAD, played hit and miss with her light therapy until she came to accept that she needed to take better care of herself. After that, everything seemed to get better and she had her best winter ever.

Sometimes taking SAD seriously means making significant life changes to ease the difficulties of everyday living during the winter. One of my patients with SAD had to spend many hours in her car each day commuting and carpooling her children, which added enormously to the daily stresses of her life and prevented her from being able to exercise regularly and get sufficient light exposure. By taking her problem seriously, she managed to persuade her husband to put their much-loved home on the market and move closer to the children's school. This life change paid off richly for the patient and her family in the ensuing winters.

Changing the Environment

More Light

The benefit of increasing environmental light can be obtained not only from formal therapy in front of a light box but also whenever your environment is brighter. Some people have several light boxes in the house, from which they can get lots of light without feeling trapped in one location. Extra light need not come only from special boxes but can be obtained by installing more lights on the ceiling or placing more lamps in the room. Once you pay attention to the amount and quality of your environmental light, you will come up with all kinds of ways to enhance it, which will help you feel more comfortable and cheerful, and give you a greater sense of control over your SAD symptoms. For more information on modifying your environment to bring more light into your life, see pages 156–158.

Winter Vacations

Many of my patients have learned that if they have a choice, it's better to take vacations in winter than in summer. Two weeks in a sunny climate in January can effectively interrupt the worst stretch of the winter. I am reminded of a television commercial in which a man stands on the beach in Jamaica looking somber on day one of his vacation. He looks a little more cheerful on day two, and is positively blissful by day three. For the SAD sufferer, this is truth in advertising! People seem to feel better in natural sunlight than they do up north, even with light therapy. As an alternative to popular seaside resorts, some of my patients have undertaken adventurous trips—for example, to Antarctica (where the days are very long when it's winter in the northern hemisphere) or the Galapagos, with similarly beneficial results.

Unfortunately, the uplifting effects of winter vacations are usually short-lived, and a regimen of light therapy must usually be resumed when you return. In some instances, people report feeling even worse after returning from a sunny climate than they did before they left the dreary weather to go on vacation. You can prevent this by restarting light therapy promptly after you return from your trip. Should depression rebound in full force, however, be sure to consult your doctor and actively step up the various elements of your self-care program.

Another cautionary note goes out to those who are overstimulated by sudden exposure to intense sunlight in the middle of winter, much as they often feel in summer. If this applies to you, when you travel to sunny places, be sure to watch out for the signs of overstimulation— loss of sleep, racing thoughts, and excessive exuberance, and decrease your exposure to sunlight if this occurs.

It should come as no surprise that a Caribbean vacation is often more uplifting than a light box perched atop a desk on a dreary New England day, but there is also a small, growing body of evidence suggesting that sunlight might affect mood via the skin as well as the eyes. One recent study described in Chapter 7 showed that tanning beds, which emit UV light, may have a euphoriant effect. Subjects in the experiment were exposed on different occasions to such beds or control tanning beds that lacked UV rays. Later, when asked to choose between these two tanning beds, most preferred the one *with* the UV rays. Other research has shown that UV rays can stimulate skin cells to secrete the chemical beta-endorphin, which produces opiate-like euphoriant effects and may explain the UV phenomenon.

Even though tanning, whether on the beach or in tanning salons, may make you cheerful, I can hardly recommend it, given its potential to cause skin cancers including the sometimes-fatal melanoma. By all means enjoy winter vacations in sunny places, but do be careful to limit direct sun exposure to the skin with sunblock and appropriate clothing (including a hat or cap).

Relocation

Several of my patients have chosen the dramatic solution of moving permanently to a place with a sunnier climate. Generally, those who have relocated feel good about their choice. They are more energetic in winter and their energy level is distributed more evenly year round. There are, of course, many factors other than climate that have to be taken into account in a decision to relocate. Besides the potential impact of lifestyle, consider the points in the box below.

SHOULD YOU RELOCATE?

- How well can your SAD symptoms be controlled by light therapy and other means?

- Will you really feel better during the winter in the new climate? One way to test this is to visit the place and see how you feel when you are there during the winter before making a commitment to move.

- What are the exact weather conditions in the place in question? For example, even though a place may be located in the South, local weather conditions may cause clouds to obscure the sun for much of the winter. You can order a booklet summarizing comparative climatic data for the United States from the National Oceanic and Atmospheric Administration in Asheville, North Carolina (call 828-271-4800 or visit *www.ncdc.noaa.gov*).

- What is the summer like in the new place, and how do you respond to heat and humidity? Be careful that a move doesn't result in exchanging one climatic problem for another.

Diet and Exercise

Diet and exercise are important for SAD sufferers, both for their valuable effect on mood and for their beneficial physical effects. People with SAD often put on weight during the winter because they eat more and exercise less. Although it is easier to lose weight during summer, there is a tendency to retain pounds with each cycle of the seasons. Over the years, these extra pounds add up and can result in obesity. Light therapy, for all its benefits, often proves disappointing to those who hope that they will automatically shed their excess weight as they begin to feel better. Diet and exercise should therefore be part of the overall health maintenance plan for people with SAD.

Exercise

There is growing evidence that regular aerobic exercise has a beneficial effect on mood control in those who suffer from depression in general. Not surprisingly, research shows that exercise is helpful for people with SAD as well.

We know that many people with SAD have increased appetite in winter. According to one study, by Siberian researcher Arcady Putilov and colleagues, they may also have slower metabolism. Aerobic exercise is known not only to burn calories but also to increase metabolism afterwards—both welcome effects for a person with SAD.

There is some evidence that combining exercise and light therapy may be more potent than either intervention alone—at least as an antidepressant (though the weight-loss potential of this combination has yet to be explored). In practice, of course, it is easy to exercise and get more light at the same time—for example, by walking briskly or jogging outdoors on a bright winter day or working out in front of a light box. Typically, people with SAD who rely on exercise alone to prevent their winter symptoms have trouble mustering the willpower to continue working out through the winter months. So the combination makes good sense. The light therapy will keep you motivated to exercise—and the exercise will be good for both mood and weight control.

In finding the best exercise regimen for you, the most important factor is finding something you enjoy—*any* exercise is better than no exercise, and if you enjoy it, you are much more likely to stick with it. If you choose the exercise on the basis of its aerobic properties or therapeutic value and don't enjoy it, it's unlikely to work out over the long haul. Finding an exercise buddy can make a big difference—you can bolster one another's motivation during the dark days. Some find it easiest to exercise as part of a group. I frequently see a group of neighborhood women out for their regular brisk morning walk, and they always seem to be having a good time. Likewise, I know several men who enjoy working out together at the gym before heading in to their jobs. If you can afford it, hiring a personal trainer may be one way to ensure that you stay with the program.

A key to losing weight is raising your metabolic rate—the rate at which you burn calories. One way to accomplish this is through vigorous exercise, especially over a sustained period, for example, 20 minutes or more. An added benefit of this "fat-burning" exercise is that you continue to burn off more calories than usual for some time after you have stopped exercising, since it takes a while for your metabolic rate to settle back down to resting levels. But remember, less vigorous exercise—such as walking round the block—will burn off calories and boost your mood too, so don't be discouraged if more intense workouts are not for you.

> *Do whatever it takes to resist the very strong temptation to be a couch potato when you have SAD and do something—anything—to keep your body active through the winter months.*

Another way that exercise can increase your metabolic rate is by replacing fat with muscle—for example, with regular weight lifting. Since muscle cells have a higher metabolic rate than fat cells, you can think of your muscles as calorie-burning factories. By increasing your muscle mass, you are also increasing the rate at which you burn calories, even at rest.

Diet and SAD

People with SAD often have a voracious appetite for foods rich in carbohydrates, such as bread, potatoes, pasta, and rice—not to mention cookies, doughnuts, and desserts—often reporting that such foods comfort them, energize them, or otherwise make them feel good. One of the problems with regulating your mood and energy with food is that the mood boost is very short-lived. Within an hour or two, the carbohydrate craver is hungry, lethargic, or irritable once more and sets out to treat this discomfort with another dose of carbohydrates.

I once believed that little could be done about these cravings. I had read that there is a set point for weight somewhere in the brain and that your body will cause you to eat more or less to ensure that you remain at that set point. Diets don't work, I was told. Biology is destiny. I was more impressed by this theory each time I stood on my bathroom scale and found my weight more or less unchanged, despite the variability in eating and exercise from day to day.

We have learned a lot about diet since those bad old days. It turns out that *what* you eat can, in fact, make a *huge* difference. The old-fashioned diets based on how many calories you eat turn out to be much more difficult to sustain than diets that emphasize where those calories come from. In the end, of course, the number of calories *does* matter—very much, in fact. But certain kinds of foods make you hungrier and therefore cause you to eat more calories. And what kinds of foods are these? You probably know them already—carbohydrates, especially high-glycemic carbohydrates.

Let me explain. All carbohydrates contain sugar molecules, which are absorbed from the bowel into the bloodstream. Once in the bloodstream, these sugar molecules cause the pancreas—a set of glands at the back of the abdomen—to secrete insulin. The insulin, in turn, pushes the glucose molecules into the tissues, such as fat storage depots, thereby lowering the blood sugar once again. Certain foods consist of carbohydrates that are rapidly dumped from the bowel into the bloodstream—they are said to have a high glycemic index and are mostly so-called simple carbohydrates. Other foods—so-called complex carbohydrates—release their sugar molecules more slowly into the bloodstream and are said to have a low glycemic index.

Foods with a high glycemic index—like candy, pasta, or potatoes—because their sugars are rapidly dumped into the bloodstream, will provoke a correspondingly dramatic increase in insulin release, which will result in a sharp drop in blood sugar. This makes you hungry again—and sets a vicious cycle in motion: bingeing (or snacking) on high-glycemic carbohydrates, yo-yo type swings in blood sugar levels, more craving, and more bingeing. And here is an even more vicious part of the cycle. As fat gets deposited, especially around the belly, as a result of all this bingeing, that fat is extra resistant to the effects of insulin. So the pancreas has to work harder and harder, secreting more and more insulin to get the blood sugar into the tissues. Finally, the pancreas begins to fail, and levels of sugar begin to build up in the blood—resulting in diabetes, which is becoming an epidemic in the United States and other developed countries.

In trying to understand the special challenges that face people with SAD, we need to think about a different twist to this cycle. As you may recall from Chapter 4, one theory about people with SAD (backed by a fair amount of data) is that they have too little serotonin in key parts of their brain during the winter—which may account for many of their symptoms, carbohydrate craving included. The insulin released by the pancreas has other actions besides pushing blood sugar into tissues. One of these actions is to push the amino acid tryptophan from the blood into the brain, where it serves as the key building block for serotonin. That may explain why people with SAD crave carbohydrates in the dark days of winter. They have somehow figured out that a handful of cookies gives them a boost in energy and mood, and when that boost passes (all too quickly), the solution is, well, another handful of cookies. In fact, one study that my colleagues and I conducted at the NIMH showed that a meal of cookies stimulated people with SAD but sedated those in the control group. One theory of how light therapy works is that it boosts brain serotonin levels in a healthier and more stable way.

As I have mentioned, the unfortunate consequence of a pattern of winter bingeing is the accumulation of body fat during the winter, some of which remains the following summer. That may explain the findings of Kurt Krauchi, Anna Wirz-Justice, and colleagues in Switzerland, who have shown that people with SAD secrete more insulin in response to a glucose load than nonseasonal controls. If patients with SAD have exaggerated insulin responses to carbohydrate-rich meals, resulting in lower than normal blood sugar levels, this could trigger cravings for more carbohydrates, and the cycle could go on and on. The Swiss researchers have found that light therapy reverses the tendency to oversecrete insulin in response to a glucose load—another possible explanation for how light therapy may reduce carbohydrate cravings.

Now millions of people have begun to realize that you can influence your weight by the *types* of food you choose to eat. There has been a nationwide shift away from carbohydrate-rich diets as a means of weight loss. Instead, diets such as the Atkins diet emphasize the benefit of limiting carbohydrates. The popular South Beach diet echoes the same theme while extolling the value of certain types of carbohydrates (complex and low glycemic) over others. In my experience, different diets work for different people. But most people with SAD need to limit their carbohydrate intake if they hope to avoid gaining weight during the winter. It is particularly important to avoid carbohydrates that consist of "empty calories"—foods that don't contain useful nutrients, such as sugar and white flour. While entire books are written about diets, let me simply outline a way of eating that has worked for me and many other carbohydrate cravers with or without SAD. You'll find additional resources on the specifics of diet and nutrition in the Resources section of the book. I would caution against extreme diets (for example, almost no carbohydrates at all). We just don't know what their potential long-term ill effects may be. We certainly don't want to exchange one health problem for another, as yet to be determined.

"Are You a Carb Craver?"

Most people with SAD crave carbohydrates in the winter and sometimes year round. As a consequence, they gain too much weight. To find out whether you are a carb craver, answer the following questions:

1.	Do you struggle to keep your weight within acceptable limits?	Yes	No
2.	Do you crave carbohydrate-rich foods like bread, cake, cookies, cereal, desserts, pretzels, sweetened sodas, fruit, or fruit juice, between meals?	Yes	No
3.	When you are eating carbohydrate-rich foods, do you have the next handful, spoonful, or forkful ready before you have finished swallowing the previous one?	Yes	No
4.	If you have had a carbohydrate-rich breakfast, do you feel hungrier in mid- to late morning than you would have had you skipped breakfast altogether or just drunk a cup of coffee that morning?	Yes	No
5.	Do you find yourself snacking on carbohydrate-rich foods between meals or after dinner at least four times per week?	Yes	No

If you answered yes to question 1 and to at least two of the four other questions, you are probably a carb craver. This is even more likely if you answered yes to more of the questions.

Some Practical Suggestions

The idea behind all carbohydrate-restricted diets is very simple: limit the amount of carbohydrate-rich foods. When you do eat carbohydrates, avoid foods that contain pure sugar, as well as white flour. That means minimizing white bread and pasta. For good measure, also minimize potatoes and white rice. What follows is a broad outline of how such a diet may play out over the course of the day.

1. Start with breakfast. For carb cravers, starting the day with the standard cereal, toast, or orange juice is a surefire way of getting your cravings going all day long. Instead, consider protein-rich alternatives.

- Eggs or egg substitutes. There are many ways to be creative with eggs so that they don't become boring.
- Fish. This could be steamed shrimp, which takes no time at all if you use the frozen type, or canned tuna or salmon. One good thing about canned salmon is that most of it is wild and free of some of the pollutants recently discovered in farm-raised salmon. Canned sardines are also good. Because they are lower on the food chain than larger fish, they are less likely to contain mercury and other pollutants.
- People vary in how much carbohydrate they can handle with breakfast, but most people with SAD find that it is important to choose the type. For example, whole wheat tortillas are a good addition. They are readily available at supermarkets and are good for a quick meal. Some people have also reported having good luck with slow-cooked steel-cut oatmeal or groats (the least-processed form of oats), which often do not trigger the degree of cravings one would expect from a carbohydrate-rich food. As always, try all these different possibilities out for yourself to see what works for you.

2. An excellent lunch is a green salad with chicken or fish. Caesar dressing is low in carbohydrates and therefore good for those whose cravings get triggered by even small amounts of sugar such as you will find in sugary vinaigrettes and other sweet dressings. For those wanting to minimize unhealthy fats and carbohydrates, pure olive oil and regular vinegar works well. In addition, nowadays entire aisles in

supermarkets are devoted to low-carbohydrate products. If you want to add small amounts of healthful carbohydrates to your salad, you can do so by sprinkling walnuts, sunflower seeds, or low-sodium whole wheat crackers over it.

3. Dinner should be a well-balanced meal containing protein, green vegetables, and fruits. Different people can get away with different amounts of carbohydrates, but, once again, try to avoid white bread and pastas. Whole wheat alternatives are preferred.

4. Snacks between meals are encouraged. Sticks of part-skim mozzarella or a handful of unsalted walnuts or almonds work well. These nuts contain omega-3 fatty acids, believed to be good for the heart and perhaps for mood as well.

5. Low-carbohydrate diets tend to be rather constipating. Salads, vegetables, and fruits tend to minimize this problem, but many people have to supplement these diets with fiber such as psyllium. Watch out for some fiber-containing supplements, which are quite caloric in their own right. If you're going to consume calories, you may as well enjoy it with high-fiber foods rather than bulk-forming laxatives.

Since I have been adhering to this type of diet, I have lost weight, gained energy, and no longer have to anticipate with horror that regular winter ritual of stepping into my trousers and finding that they no longer fit. Best of all, the cravings have gone and I no longer feel as though I am constantly deprived. Many of my patients have had similar good luck, so I pass these observations on to you in the hope that you too will find them useful.

Remember, no diet is right for everybody. There are many different kinds of diets out there, and many good books on the subject. If you have special needs, such as those posed by diabetes, you would do well to consult with a dietitian or your doctor to be sure that the diet you choose is right for you.

To Weigh or Not to Weigh?: That Is the Question

It seems as though there are two types of people: those who like to weigh themselves and those who don't. I fall into the first group. Any scientist knows that to find out the results of an experiment, you have to measure something, and when it comes to a diet, that measurement is weight. For people with SAD, the pounds can sneak on relentlessly throughout the winter unless you keep an eye on the scale, and increases in weight invariably lead to drops in mood. If you are one of those people who likes to know how much they weigh, I recommend that you weigh yourself daily *and write down your weight.* That way you can establish a baseline and find out what causes your weight to go up or down. Then, when you start a diet, you can sort out the effects of the diet from the weight fluctuations that occur from day to day or across the month. You can set realistic goals for yourself and see where you are in relation to them.

Some people really hate to weigh themselves. Doing so may cause them to obsess about their weight and may not be good for them. For that reason, the question of whether to weigh yourself (and how frequently) has to be an individual judgment.

Meditation: Help from an Unexpected Source

In Chapter 11 we will consider the novel possibility that meditation might actually help people with SAD. As you will see, I became interested in the topic because of my own experience with one form of meditation, Transcendental Meditation (TM), which was very helpful to me personally. That inspired me to recommend meditation to various patients. The reason for my raising the topic here as well is that after starting to meditate, I experienced a slow loss of weight (about 8 pounds), which happened over many months and, surprisingly, it stayed off. Since the meditation was the only new factor in the equation, I suspected that it might be the explanation for the weight loss. Many people, myself included, eat when stressed. Since meditation is known to reduce stress, that might be how it could promote weight loss.

I encouraged my weight loss and fitness expert, Pamela Peeke, to learn TM as well. Impressed by the ability of the technique to reduce stress, Peeke also recommended meditation to patients—with excellent results. Peeke describes her findings in her book "The Hunger Fix" (see Resource section). Somehow, reducing stress helps people stay grounded and moderate their eating behavior. After reading Chapter 11, you might consider including some form of meditation into your SAD management program.

Herbs, Vitamins, and Supplements

You need look no further than your daily papers to find advertisements for herbs, vitamins, and supplements for all sorts of ailments, including SAD. It is important to sort out fact from fiction (or conjecture) as these supplements can be expensive and are not necessarily harmless. So, what can truthfully be said in favor of supplements for SAD—or supplements in general? People ask me, "What do you take?" understandably wanting to know my bottom line conclusions. So, here they are:

- Fish oil extracts (concentrates of omega-3 fatty acids)—2 grams per day
- Calcium citrate—1,260 milligrams per day
- Vitamin D_3—5,000 units/day (highly variable from person to person)
- Multivitamin—1 per day

You can make excellent arguments for many other vitamins and supplements. I have done so myself and tried to stay ahead of the curve, taking L-carnitine and alpha-lipoic acid, resveratrol, N-acetylcysteine, and many other substances. In the end, however, I was not persuaded of their effectiveness, and got tired of gobbling handfuls of expensive pills. In defense of N-acetylcysteine, I should say there is some evidence that it may be helpful in people susceptible to bipolar depression.

Wondering whether my relatively modest regimen of supplements was reasonable, I checked in with my friend and colleague Mehmet Oz, cardiovascular surgeon and star of *The Dr. Oz Show*. I was pleased to find that his own personal daily regimen was quite similar to my own.

Omega-3 fatty acids may be helpful for cardiac function and may have a beneficial effect on both depression and bipolar disorder. I say "may have" because the data are mixed, and some of the best studies of omega fatty acids for depression have been negative.

Many people in the United States are deficient Vitamin D_3, an enormously important vitamin. One reason for the drop in D levels is that most of us now use sunscreen (appropriately so) to block the sun's UV rays. These rays, however, are responsible for vitamin D synthesis in the skin. So protecting the skin from sunburn and skin cancer can also render us deficient in this essential vitamin. One good thing about vitamin D is that it can be readily measured in the blood and you can determine whether your levels are in the approved range. If not, simply take enough so that you get there. The amount of vitamin D present in ordinary multivitamin tablets will probably be far too little to do the job.

Some people have suggested that vitamin D may itself be an antidepressant for people with SAD. Evidence for this is purely anecdotal. Some individuals swear that it has helped them, and small uncontrolled studies have been encouraging. So far, however, there have been no controlled studies of this question. The theory behind this line of research is that the lack of sunlight in winter causes vitamin D deficiency, which in turn causes the symptoms of SAD. If this were correct (and for now, there is no evidence to support this theory), then replacing the missing vitamin D might also improve mood.

There may be a place for other vitamins as well in the treatment of SAD. The most compelling case for the role of vitamins in treating depression in general involves vitamin B_1 (thiamine): four separate controlled studies found a mood-elevating effect for 50 milligrams per day. Other B vitamins such as B_{12} and folic acid may also be helpful. I outline the case for vitamins in treating depression in my 2002 book *The Emotional Revolution: How the New Science of Feelings Can Transform Your Life*.

St. John's Wort

There are many studies suggesting that St. John's wort, an extract of a flowering herb, is an active antidepressant. Some of my patients take it with good effects. One problem with using St. John's wort in people with SAD is that it is a known photosensitizer—which means that when sunlight hits tissues (skin or eyes) of people taking the herb they can experience side effects, such as painful sunburn or eye pains. In fact, several members of SADA, the SAD Association of Great Britain, who undertook a trial of St. John's wort for SAD complained of painful eyes when they used the herbal extract together with their usual light therapy. Although it is unclear whether any actual harm resulted from this combination, the presence of these symptoms is discouraging, and

I do not recommend the concomitant use of St. John's wort and light therapy at this time.

For those seeking to use the herb, usual dosages range from 300 to 1,800 milligrams per day. Besides photosensitization, side effects include irritability, insomnia, and decreased sexual responsiveness.

Watch Out for Alcohol and Marijuana

Alcohol tends to make depressed people even more depressed. True, you may get an initial buzz that may even carry you through an evening, but in many cases depressed people will pay dearly for this in the form of lowered mood and energy over the next few days. This warning applies even more strongly against marijuana, which can increase depression and sap you of much-needed motivation and is notorious for causing "the munchies." Also, contrary to popular belief, marijuana can be quite addictive. In discussions with many colleagues, I have encountered concerns similar to my own about the downside of marijuana, especially for people with mood disorders.

Stress Management

If you are a seasonal person, you have the advantage of being able to predict that at some times of the year your energy level will be low and it may be difficult to get certain things done that at other times of the year may be a snap. You can use this information to regulate your stress level throughout the year. Although some stresses are unpredictable and cannot be planned for, many can be anticipated—such as buying a new house, moving, starting a new job, and taking on a writing deadline. Beware of setting spring deadlines and delivery dates on projects. A common trap when you are riding high during the summer is to promise to complete a project within 9 months, which may seem ample, only to end up struggling to meet your overoptimistic projection when your energy level sinks to its lowest winter ebb.

Many people use the summer months for the creative aspects of their work and the winter months to consolidate and work on more humdrum tasks. Our original seasonal patient, Herb Kern, adopted this pattern. An engineer at a large laboratory, he had his best ideas and conducted his most exciting experiments in summer, then wrote up his data—a more routine task—in winter. Some famous composers, most notably Handel and Mahler, were seasonal and did most of their composing in the summer months.

Chapter 12, "A Step-by-Step Guide through the Revolving Year," will give you ideas as to how you can look over your year in its entirety and plan accordingly.

One way to reduce stress in winter is to pay for help and services. You can use some of that money you are not spending for the type of socializing and shopping you do in the summer to pay others for help with difficult chores such as taking your clothes to the laundry, cleaning your house, or buying takeout dinners. Mothers can have a particularly hard time meeting the demands of small children when they are feeling depressed, and paying for extra child or home care can provide a great deal of relief. If you have some money to spare, think of ways to solve a problem by hiring someone else to do chores, such as grocery shopping and housekeeping. You may find yourself coming up with some rather creative solutions.

Sometimes feelings of guilt can be an obstacle to getting the help you need. In that case, remind yourself that you are not being lazy, neglectful, and all the other negative adjectives that depressed people are so good at using on themselves. Reduced levels of energy and motivation—and inability to cope—are key symptoms of depression. Even though you may be doing many things to reduce these symptoms, these measures may not be completely effective. It is therefore very important to reduce your stresses and commitments, and if paying others to help out is financially possible, it is worth doing so for the sake of your mental health. Remember, too, that paying someone to take care of certain chores may give you more time and energy to devote to your job, and it is false economy to skimp on help with chores if your job is at stake.

A major problem for depressed people is concentrating and remembering. Many seasonal people have developed methods of coping with these difficulties. One woman I know has developed some tricks to help her remember things in the winter. For example, she records everything on her calendar and doesn't assume that she will remember things that she would recall easily in the summertime. She cross-indexes the people she relies on for help of various kinds under a section labeled "H" for "Help." This section includes addresses and phone numbers of plumbers, workmen, and even her doctors, whose names she often forgets in the winter. She leaves notes for herself on the back door, where she will see them as she goes out of the house, and writes notes to herself late at night about what she needs to do the following morning. She also writes down other information, such as friends' birthdays and directions to people's homes.

For many older patients with SAD, retirement offers a particular type of relief from stress. One such gentleman who had worked for many years as an architect said, "I have been free of all SAD symptoms for the past 3 years since I retired, and I recommend it to everyone." Retirement, like relocation, is a major life decision that involves many considerations, including the loss of a meaningful job, reduced income, and having to structure the days that were previously filled up with work. The dilemma was articulated by a couple who consulted me about how best to manage the wife's SAD symptoms. She had been a head nurse on a busy unit for many years and was having increasing difficulties functioning effectively during the winter. Her husband, also a professional and very supportive of her, was concerned that she would feel even worse if she lost the daily structure that her work afforded her. When I suggested that the work appeared to offer more stress than comfort, the wife expressed great relief. Quitting her job or giving up the head nurse position would give her more control over her hours—and that might make a critical difference to her comfort level. Once he became aware of how she felt about the matter, the husband pointed out that they would have more than enough money to enable her to stop working and supported her decision.

> As far as stress management is concerned, the bottom line is nurture your resources and use your creativity to find shortcuts and ways to conserve your energy that will help keep you going through the down season.

Negative Ions

As I mentioned earlier in the book, positively charged particles in the air, also known as "positive ions," have long been regarded as mentally disturbing to those in their path. These positive ions are swept along at high density by "ill winds," such as the hot Santa Ana winds in California, which, as writer Raymond Chandler so aptly put it, sent housewives reaching for their kitchen knives while eyeing the backs of their husbands' necks. An old, patchy literature suggested a remedy for the unsettling effects of such ill winds: exposure to negatively charged particles, also known as "negative ions." A negative ion generator would shift the balance of ambient negative to positive ions in a favorable direction. As you may recall, negative ions occur in nature near waterfalls, the pounding surf, or after a rainstorm—environments where we often feel good. Research now shows that there might be some genuine scientific basis to this idea.

Michael and Jiuan Su Terman at Columbia Psychiatric Institute rigorously tested the effects of negative ions on patients with SAD. They found that sitting in front of a machine that puts out a flow of negative ions at a high rate (a negative ion generator) for 30 minutes each morning for a week produces as powerful an antidepressant effect as sitting in front of a 10,000-lux light box for the same duration. The high-flow-rate ion generator maintains a high density of ions in the room. A control negative ion generator calibrated to put out only a low flow rate of negative ions (low-density ion generator) was vastly inferior, no better than a placebo. The results of the Termans' first study were exciting but preliminary. Scientists always like to see results replicated before getting really excited. Well, the Termans went on to replicate their original findings, but with a slight twist. This time they administered the negative ions to patients with SAD during the last 45 to 90 minutes of sleep. To ensure that the ions really went to the patients and not to the radiator and other grounded structures in the room, the Termans connected the ion generator to a grounded sheet on which their subjects slept. Once again, the high-density ion generator turned out to be roughly as effective as light therapy (30 minutes at 10,000 lux) and vastly superior to a low-density control generator. So far, no side effects have emerged; nor is there any theoretical reason to expect side effects since we routinely encounter high densities of negative ions under natural circumstances. I have had good luck with the ion generator, at least in one person with SAD who had tried many other forms of treatment with limited success. Yet, in his case, the addition of the ion generator appeared to make an important difference. So, if you are looking for yet another approach to treat your SAD, you may seriously want to consider obtaining a high-output negative ion generator.

One caveat: The Termans caution against using a light box and an ion generator simultaneously as the ion flow could be diverted to the grounded light box.

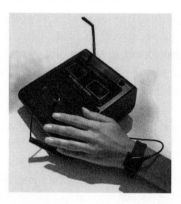

No medications, no effort, no side effects! It sounds too good to be true—especially since we have no idea how the ion generator may work. But that is what the data suggest. So, expect to see a lot more about negative ions in the years to come.

Meanwhile, you can try this novel treatment for yourself simply by purchasing and plugging in the ion generator shown in Figure 8 (the manufacturer is listed in the Resources) and switching it on and off next to your bed with the help of a standard silent electronic timer.

FIGURE 8. The negative ion generator available from the Center for Environmental Therapeutics. Photo by John Kristoffersen.

Support Groups

Support groups have been helpful to people with all sorts of problems. Members of such groups join forces for many reasons, including:

- Sharing the latest information, tips, and inspirational stories
- Working toward common goals—such as universal insurance reimbursement for light therapy devices
- Having group sessions where people can meet and offer help and hope to one another

The only SAD support group with a sustained track record of effectiveness is the highly successful Seasonal Affective Disorder Association of Great Britain (SADA), which has answered hundreds of thousands of queries over its decades of operation, has regular annual meetings, and raises money for research into the condition. This group, which has done an enormous amount of good for people with SAD in the United Kingdom, has relied heavily on a small core of dedicated volunteers. In addition, its existence would not have been possible without the indefatigable perseverance of its founder, Jennifer Eastwood.

Certainly there is a need for the same type of group in this country. Millions of people are suffering from the condition, relevant new scientific and technical advances are being made regularly, and the public has a tremendous need for support and up-to-date information about SAD and its treatment. With a relatively small core of effective volunteers, it might be possible to found and maintain a vibrant SAD support group. That would be a highly worthwhile project for someone with interest in this particular cause.

One problem that a SAD support group faces is that all its members tend to be at their lowest ebb at the same time—during the winter—just when there is the greatest need for information and support. For this reason, it would be a good idea to hire an unaffected person or recruit friends and relatives of those with SAD, who could keep a support group running during the dark days.

Acceptance

Sometimes, even with the best therapy, mood control is not perfect. As long as the lows are not too low or too long, a measure of acceptance can sometimes be very therapeutic. Many of us expect to function happily and at peak levels at all times. By expecting this, we often place unreasonable demands on ourselves, which require machine-like efficiency. A great measure of contentment can be attained by accepting as inevitable some degree of fluctuation in energy, mood, and ability to function as part of the ordinary ebb and flow of life. This concept is more in keeping with Eastern than Western thinking. For example, the ancient Chinese medical guide, the *Nei Ching*, advises people to behave in certain specific ways during each season, recommending, for example, that during winter people should go to bed early and arise late. The message is to yield to the physical and emotional changes that come with the changing seasons rather than to oppose them. After you have done all you can to reverse the unpleasant and disabling symptoms of SAD, that is not bad advice. You will find more about Eastern approaches to dealing with stress and suffering in the chapter on meditation (Chapter 11).

Acceptance often comes slowly, bit by bit, rather than all at once. There is a great temptation each year, as spring arrives, to think that the problem is over, only to have it reappear again the following fall. That can be annoying, frustrating, and, in itself, depressing. For example, one woman with a 15-year history of SAD has been treated with light therapy, antidepressant medications, and psychotherapy with considerable success. Her depressions no longer disable her as they once did, but she is still less energetic, enthusiastic, and effective in the winter than in the summer. Last winter, for the first time, she felt enraged at the limitations the condition imposes on her, the way her life seems to flip-flop between feeling good and feeling depressed every 6 months. This anger is one more phase in her slow journey toward acceptance.

To summarize, there are many different approaches you can take to help yourself cope with winter depression and turn a previously dreaded season into a time of joy. A first step requires the recognition that the difficulties associated with depression—low energy level, pessimism, lack of motivation, low self-esteem, and withdrawal, to name just a few—are symptoms of an illness, not flaws in your character. They require understanding rather than judgment and condemnation, serious attention rather than denial and minimization, and the first person who needs to understand them and take them seriously is the depressed person. This is helpful in itself. In addition, for people with seasonal depression, changing the environment may be quite beneficial. Brighten your living and work areas, travel to sunny places in the winter, or, if all else fails, relocate permanently to a better climate.

Exercise moderately and regularly in a way you find enjoyable. Find a companion to join you, and help each other stick to your routine. Diet sensibly and consider a low-carbohydrate diet. Limit stresses. Don't make commitments during your summer highs that you are unable to keep in the winter. Anticipate predictable chores and use your creativity to figure out solutions ahead of time. Stay informed. New treatments and devices, such as negative ion generators, are being discovered all the time—and yesterday's unsolvable problem may have a solution today. If you're the kind of person who derives comfort from others who are in a situation similar to yours, join a support group of fellow sufferers—or establish your own! Finally, *accept* that which you cannot change. Life has its ups and downs, and no one understands that better than the SAD sufferer. But before resigning yourself to your problems, be sure that you have explored all the treatments outlined in this book, including psychotherapy and antidepressant medications, which I discuss in the next two chapters, and possibly meditation as well, covered in Chapter 11.

NINE

Psychotherapy and SAD

▶ How do you decide when to seek therapy?

▶ If you've decided to enter therapy, what sort should you seek?

▶ How do you find and choose a therapist?

    ▶ How do you know whether you can trust a particular therapist to treat your deepest and most private thoughts and feelings with respect?

    ▶ How do you know whether the therapist is competent, will understand your problem, and will know the appropriate thing to say or do about it?

▶ How do you integrate psychotherapy with light therapy or antidepressant medications?

▶ How do you know whether the therapy is working?

For many people with seasonal difficulties psychotherapy may be helpful, but it is by no means universally necessary. If you're considering psychotherapy for SAD, this chapter provides an overview of the topic. For more information, see the Resources.

When Should You Consider Entering Therapy?

Suppose you suffer from winter depressions. You seek out a therapist qualified to treat you with light therapy or antidepressant medications and find that this takes care of many, if not all, of your symptoms. In addition, you take steps to embrace a positive lifestyle as outlined elsewhere in this book. You now have an explanation for your seasonal difficulties and, moreover, a way to treat and control them. This frees you to get on with your life, to love and to work, as Freud would say, and also to enjoy yourself. Do you need psychotherapy? Of course not.

Now imagine a different scenario. Your seasonal symptoms have responded to treatment. You no longer sink to the depths of depression familiar to you for so many years. All should be well, but it is not. Something is amiss. Perhaps you feel stuck where you are in life. You have been following certain routines and activities that once were fulfilling but now are not. Some change is necessary, but nothing suggests itself to you. Persisting in the same course gets you nowhere in this mission. Or perhaps you feel trapped in certain gloomy ways of viewing yourself or the world around you. At this point, psychotherapy can be beneficial. It can help you define the problem and search within yourself for solutions that may be very difficult to find on your own.

Melissa, a public relations professional in her early 40s, is an example of the second sort of person. Intelligent, talented, attractive, with a charming personality, she nonetheless grew up believing that she was a failure. It was not difficult to trace this painful set of beliefs to her parents—both college professors who had not accomplished all that they had hoped to do. They had not made seminal original contributions, nor had they won any international awards. They invested their hopes in Melissa to do this in their stead. Unfortunately for them, Melissa had neither the talent nor the inclination to meet these expectations. Although she defiantly set out to chart her own course in life both personally and professionally, deep down she never felt good enough. This core sense of inadequacy played itself out both at work—where she rarely asked for the raises and promotions she might easily have been given—and in her personal life. She felt inadequate as a wife and mother, even though others generally viewed her as extremely competent.

After entering the seasonal program at the NIMH and having her winter depression treated with light therapy, Melissa embarked on a course of psychotherapy. Through this process she was able to understand how she had been programmed to believe she was never good enough. Therefore, no matter what she did, or how successful she was, it didn't feel adequate. She was not fulfilling that early programming and her parents' expectations. Once she understood the origins of her feelings of failure—her parents' unfair and unrealistic expectations of her—she was able to better define her expectations for herself and recognize that these new expectations—her own—were both legitimate and compatible with what she truly wanted to do with her life. Psychotherapy was a liberating experience for her. Whereas light therapy reversed the symptoms of her winter depression, psychotherapy helped her understand and come to terms with problems from her past— something that light therapy by itself could not have accomplished.

I have seen many people besides Melissa achieve successful and liberating effects from good psychotherapy. I have also seen psychotherapy and other forms of treatment work well together, as they did for Melissa. If you have significant problems like Melissa's that persist after treatment with light therapy or medications, you should certainly consider psychotherapy.

Cognitive-Behavioral Therapy for SAD

Of all types of psychotherapy for SAD, cognitive-behavioral therapy (CBT) has the most going for it. Not only do studies provide evidence for its effectiveness specifically for SAD, but these results are buttressed by a huge literature showing that CBT is effective for depression in general. For people who do not choose to use light therapy or antidepressants, CBT alone may be sufficient for successfully treating SAD. What does this amazing treatment consist of and how can you incorporate its principles into your daily life to combat the symptoms of depression even without a therapist? For answers to these questions, read on.

There are still many people who believe that the way to resolve an emotional problem is to probe for some hidden sorrow, uncover it,

> The mind can be divided into three parts: what we think, what we feel, and what we do—or, in psychological terms, cognition, emotion, and behavior. All problems of the psyche result from disturbances in one or more of these domains or in some disconnect between them. All efforts to treat these disturbances involve tinkering with one or more of these domains or with the connection between them.

and, in so doing, resolve it. Though there may still be a role for such an approach in certain situations, the proponents of CBT take a completely different tack. They deal with what is readily apparent in cognition, emotion, and behavior. They examine the conscious (surface) thoughts related to these three domains and their relationships to one another and seek to alter or correct any apparent disturbances. In the words of Aaron Beck, one of the pioneers of CBT, there is more to the surface than meets the eye.

To their immense credit, CBT researchers have developed standardized ways of conceptualizing problems of cognition, emotion, and behavior and standardized ways to help fix them. These methods can be explained in terms readily understandable to the depressed person and can be implemented in therapy. You might be surprised at how much progress you can make by implementing the principles of CBT on your own. But even those undergoing CBT under the guidance of a therapist are urged to do homework between sessions. This emphasis on homework is soundly based on both behavioral observations and basic brain science.

Both the Beck Institute for Cognitive Behavior Therapy and the Academy of Cognitive Therapy maintain websites where you can locate a certified cognitive therapist in your area (see the Resources section).

Practice, Practice, Practice

It is a commonplace that practice makes perfect, but true nonetheless. That golf swing, video game, or piano fugue you are trying to master, the new language you would love to speak, your bridge, Scrabble, or chess game will improve by only one means: practice. So it is with all skills. To improve, you have to practice them. CBT therapists typically assign written homework in which they ask patients to record their feelings, thoughts, and actions. In depression these all typically take on a gloomy turn. The therapist teaches the patient to question these downers and turn them into uppers instead. An old song exhorts the listener to accentuate the positive and eliminate the negative. It sounds simplistic. Amazingly, though, it works, but only through continuous repetition.

Brain imaging techniques show that practice expands that portion of the brain involved in carrying out the task in question. Violinists, for example, who use their left hands to form the notes that make their music, show expansion in parts of the brain responsible for orchestrating the movements of the left hand. In contrast, those brain parts that govern the right hand, which violinists use to move their bows up and down, a far simpler task, show no such expansion. London cab drivers, who are required to learn the location of all of London's many streets to get their licenses, grow that part of their brain responsible for spatial memory.

Although it may take a violinist years to master his or her art, it is not necessary for practice to occur over such a long period for it to change the brain. On the contrary, humans and other primates taught simple skills over the course of days undergo changes in those parts of the brain responsible for the skills. New connections between nerve cells are forged, and the brain regions involved actually grow. It is a wonder to contemplate the brain, this intricate mass of mortal coils, actually growing and changing throughout adult life. For this change to be purposeful, however, practice needs to be guided. We need a teacher, coach, or mentor to show us what we are doing wrong and how to fix it. We need to learn new methods, implement them, and practice, practice, practice. That is how CBT therapists approach the treatment of depression, and they have evidence to back up their recommendations.

Brain changes in depressed patients following a course of CBT have been shown through the use of brain imaging techniques by Helen Mayberg (Professor of Psychiatry and Neurology at Emory University) and her colleagues. Specifically, certain cortical areas that may contribute to the chatter of negative thoughts quiet down after CBT, while core parts of the emotional brain become more active after therapy. These results suggest that CBT causes changes in those brain regions involved in attention and memory and that those changes drive the antidepressant response. These findings are consistent with the idea that CBT involves "top down" processing whereby patients learn to short-circuit their negative thinking patterns, as measured by decreased activity in certain cortical or "top" regions, and that this boosts mood, as measured by increased activity in the emotional or "bottom" regions.

CBT versus Light Therapy

There are by now so many studies showing the benefits of light therapy for SAD that it seems like a given that light is an effective treatment for this condition. Yet it took 14 years from our first controlled study of light therapy before the field as a whole definitively accepted this treatment, and, for all I know, there may still be some die-hard skeptics out there. In contrast, to date there have been only two studies of CBT for SAD. Preliminary results are so encouraging, however, that they are definitely worth a good look, especially since they lead to specific steps that people with SAD can take to alleviate their suffering.

The studies in question were the brainchild of Kelly Rohan, now an associate professor of psychology at the University of Vermont. While at the Uniformed Services University of the Health Sciences in Bethesda, Maryland, Rohan first compared three different forms of treatment for people with SAD: conventional light therapy, CBT, and a combination of the two treatments. In a study of 23 people with SAD, she found all three treatments to be similarly effective. Encouraged by these preliminary results, Rohan embarked on a larger study of 61 people with SAD, comparing the same three treatments—light therapy, CBT, and CBT combined with light therapy—versus a wait-list control group. As in the first study, all three active conditions were similarly effective and were all more effective than the wait-list condition. Rohan's most interesting findings however emerged the winter after the initial study. In a follow-up of participants from both studies, Rohan found that significantly more people who had been treated exclusively with light therapy (36.7%) relapsed the next winter as compared with those who had received CBT as part (5.5%) or all (7%) of their treatment. People treated with CBT alone, but not those treated with the combination treatment, also had less severe depressive symptoms the next winter compared to those treated with light therapy alone.

As best I can understand, the likely explanation for this distinction is that with light treatment alone the researchers encouraged patients to focus only on the light therapy and not at all on their lives. With CBT, on the other hand, they encouraged participants to work hard to change their thoughts and behavior during the winter and thereby to improve the quality of their lives. I have long encouraged the latter approach, as you can tell from the contents of this book. An active, even aggressive, attitude toward your SAD symptoms and winter is best. Many elements in this book echo those in Rohan's program: pursuing positive thoughts and activities and avoiding negative ones, keeping active, and interacting with people who lift your spirits. But in addition to these recommendations, Rohan's program borrows from classical CBT teachings to include specific elements that are part of what CBT is all about. Let us now examine the essentials of Rohan's program. Afterward, let's explore some specific CBT techniques.

Rohan's Anti-SAD CBT Program

Rohan conducted her program in a group setting over 6 weeks, offering two sessions each week. Here are the key elements of a CBT program such as hers that you can try out for yourself.

1. Educate yourself about SAD.
2. Consider how your activities contribute to your SAD symptoms.
3. Seek out pleasant activities.
4. Consider how your thoughts contribute to your SAD symptoms.
5. Correct erroneous thought patterns (cognitive distortions).
6. Identify themes in your negative thinking.
7. Challenge your core negative beliefs about yourself.
8. Maintain your gains and work to prevent relapse.

Self-Education: SAD as a Vicious Cycle

The more you know about SAD, the better equipped you will be to deal with and overcome it. You will find in the pages of this book much of what you need to know to do so. One important point that

Rohan stresses is how SAD can be a vicious cycle. Some SAD behaviors actually make SAD symptoms worse, which in turn aggravates those very same behaviors. For example, sleeping late prevents you from taking in the early morning light, which makes your SAD (and oversleeping) worse. Likewise people with SAD often avoid social engagements, which further isolates and depresses them.

Think of the behaviors that contribute to your SAD symptoms and write them down in a special homework log.

Seeking Out Pleasant Activities

Pleasant activities by definition elevate your mood. Make a list of those activities that give your mood a boost and push yourself to do them even if they don't come easily to you. Plan ahead by making an appointment with yourself to do a specific activity, even scheduling it into your daily planner for a specific day and at a specific time, to increase the chance that you will follow through. That way you will be less likely to back out of an activity that may improve your mood.

Remember, these activities can be pursued either indoors or outdoors. Most people can find something that will propel them out of hibernation mode. Think hard and find your own mood-boosting activities. In my own case, that means pushing myself to go walking first thing in the morning (with the help of a friend if necessary) and throwing myself into the whirl of holiday socializing even if I don't always relish the prospect. My reward: more energy during the day and an enjoyable sense of being connected with congenial people.

Rohan urges her study participants to make a commitment to pursuing pleasant activities. Analyze what is preventing you from having fun and remove all obstacles. You can do this, for example, by being sure you put enjoyable pursuits high on your priority list. Plan ahead to ensure that you get work and chores done to allow you time for joyful or spiritually uplifting activities.

Once again, make a list, keep a log of what works, and practice doing it, even if it is only for 10 minutes a day. Remember, what you practice repeatedly changes the structure and function of your brain and shapes the quality of your life. In the words of the writer Annie Dillard, "How we spend our days is of course how we spend our lives."

Understanding How Your Thoughts Affect Your Mood

One of Aaron Beck's great insights was the recognition that our thoughts affect our moods. By changing your thoughts you can change your mood with positive results.

This profound insight may seem obvious now, but it was by no means so several decades ago when I was training to become a psychiatrist. Although psychiatrists recognized that depressed people had gloomy thoughts, many concluded that these were an irreducible part of the clinical picture that would resist any reasoned attempts to alter them. By their research studies, Beck and his colleagues disproved that notion. They observed that in depressed people negative thoughts flow automatically and these automatic negative thoughts (or ANTs, as they are often called) can be identified and altered. The acronym "ANTs" calls to mind ants crawling all over one's brain—not a pleasant image but one that might readily conjure up a counterimage of oneself as exterminator, systematically getting rid of them.

CBT therapists talk of the A-B-C model, in which A stands for the *antecedent* event, B for the *belief* (or ANT) that this event produces, and C for the *consequence* of the event, or the emotion it produces. In depressed people, things often happen to make them feel worse. What CBT encourages you to do is to catch the intervening thought, between the event and the feeling, and work on changing that thought. Many research studies have shown that disputing depressed thinking, or ANTs, can elevate mood. So, D for *dispute* is added to the A-B-C mnemonic to suggest the therapeutic remedy for this toxic sequence of thoughts and feelings.

How does the A-B-C model play out in practice? Consider the example of Jack, who is turned down by a young lady when he calls her up for a date. That knocks him into a tailspin. He believes he is unattractive and undesirable to women and will never find a soul mate. These unbidden gloomy thoughts (ANTs) flood his mind and plunge him into a profound state of morbid pessimism and despair. Jack is an excellent candidate for CBT, as the sections that follow reveal. He should keep a log of his negative thoughts each day and try to understand what triggers them and how they affect his mood. He should be encouraged to act as a researcher, to investigate the workings of his own mind as a basis for addressing his problems.

Here is the type of dialogue that a CBT therapist might encourage Jack to practice both in therapy sessions and on his own.

THERAPIST: What evidence is there that she finds you unattractive and undesirable?

JACK: She turned down my invitation.

THERAPIST: Other than finding you unattractive and undesirable, why might she have declined your invitation?

[It is important to acknowledge that the ANT is one possible explanation for the woman's behavior, but to explore plausible alternative explanations.]

THERAPIST: Let's assume that this one woman really does find you unattractive and undesirable. So what? Could you live with that?

JACK: It will hurt, but probably I could.

THERAPIST: Have there been any past instances when other women behaved as though they found you desirable or attractive?

[Jack must now collect evidence against his beliefs that all women will find him unattractive and undesirable and reject him.]

THERAPIST: What qualities do you look for in a partner?

[This is an important question because it emphasizes that we all have qualities we look for in a mate, Jack included. It also helps him question whether he has been seeking out the right kind of woman for himself. After all, the right kind of mate is one who likes *you*.]

THERAPIST: Have you ever declined an invitation for a date?

JACK: Well, yes, I have on a few occasions.

THERAPIST: Why was that?

JACK: I just didn't find the one woman appealing, and the other one was loud and unkind. I saw her shouting at her little sister in the mall.

THERAPIST: It seems as though those women didn't feel like good matches for you. Obviously, matches are a two-way street and they have to feel right for both parties.

JACK: I guess you're right.

THERAPIST: What qualities do you think women are looking for in a partner?

JACK: Good looks, kindness, the ability to earn a decent income.

THERAPIST: How do you feel you stack up on those qualities?

JACK: Well, I'm not a bad-looking guy, and I'm a nice guy, but I don't have much money.

THERAPIST: Can you imagine some woman out there being interested in someone who is good-looking and kind even if he doesn't have that much money right now?

JACK: I guess.

THERAPIST: What's the worst thing that could happen with your love life?

JACK: That nobody will ever want to date me again.

THERAPIST: That is an important ANT for you to think about because if you hold on to it too firmly, it could become a self-fulfilling prophecy. It's an ideal type of ANT for us to work on. What's the best thing you can imagine happening in your love life?

JACK: Finding Ms. Right tomorrow and living happily ever after.

THERAPIST: Okay, let's look at the likelihood of these two different extreme scenarios. Rate the likelihood that each will happen on a scale of zero to 100.

[Sometimes it is useful to look at extremes to recognize that the most likely scenario lies somewhere in the middle. It's a way of bringing home the fact that in the dating game—and in life in general—there are hits and misses but that perseverance pays off in finding a compatible partner with whom to lead a good life.]

THERAPIST: What else would you like to achieve in your life, other than finding a soul mate? How are you doing in each of these areas?

[This sort of question is very useful as it broadens one's thinking about what is important in life and how you define your worth in your own mind. It is important also to point out that romantic love is only one kind of love and that the love of family and friends is also important and can bring feelings of closeness and satisfaction.]

As you can see, it really helps to have a trained therapist asking the right questions and keeping you on task. But whether or not you have such a therapist, consider keeping a daily log of your thoughts and feelings and see if you can identify which thoughts lead to negative beliefs that lower your mood. Nail down the A-B-C sequence in your own life as a necessary prelude to D, disputing and challenging this sequence and thereby improving your spirits.

Recognizing Different Types of Cognitive Distortions

CBT therapists have ingeniously categorized cognitive distortions in a very helpful way. Jack displays three types of cognitive distortions: *overgeneralization, magnification (catastrophizing)*, and *fortune-telling*. He blows the episode out of proportion and, generalizing from this single event, concludes that he is universally undesirable. Then he looks into his crystal ball and predicts that he will live out a life of lonely isolation. He considers these thoughts to be the only possible way of viewing that one event, being turned down by the young lady. He doesn't consider any other explanations for her behavior or other possible future scenarios for himself. She may be involved with another man or woman. Her cat might have died the previous day. Or she may not be interested in him, but another woman might find him irresistible.

The CBT therapist would teach him to diagnose the nature of his cognitive distortions and help him dispute them and ask "What other reasons may there be for her rejection?" and "What other outcomes can you envision other than a life of unremitting misery and loneliness?" That might then result in new behaviors that would help correct the cognitive distortion and glum forecasting, such as asking another woman out on a date (or another ten women, if necessary). After all, the young man in question is seeking only one fine lady. So what difference does it make if he finds her on the first try or on the eleventh?

Let us now consider other types of distortions. Janet receives a B+ on a term paper in an important course. When she sees the grade on the paper, her heart sinks. She believes that it represents a shockingly bad performance and that her professor, for whom she has the highest regard, must despise her for it. She had worked hard to maintain an A average throughout the semester and now regards herself as a failure who will bring shame on her parents, who have scrimped and saved to put her through school. "I must do better next time," she tells herself. "I just have to, or I will be doomed to be a failure for the rest of my life."

Janet is engaging in several types of cognitive distortion: *black-or-white thinking, magnification (catastrophizing), minimization, mind reading, fortune-telling, labeling,* and *"should" statements.* She sees her performance in black-or-white terms: either as wonderful or terrible. She doesn't consider that a B grade on the paper might be quite good when assigned by a strict professor. She magnifies the importance of the grade out of all proportion and minimizes her performance on other elements in the course. Perhaps the paper counts for only a percentage of the final grade, and even if it pulls her grade down to a B, that might be very respectable. And that one class may count for very little when viewed as part of her larger transcript. A skillful CBT therapist will encourage Janet to ask the right questions: "Do I have to see this single event in black-or-white terms? Am I making a mountain out of a molehill? Am I minimizing other aspects of my performance? How else might I view this development?"

Furthermore, Janet is engaging in *mind reading* when she jumps to the conclusion that her professor must think poorly of her. She might ask instead, "How else might he view me?" and "Even if he does not regard this particular effort as stellar, how much difference will that make in the long run [or even short run]?" Janet is also engaging in *fortune-telling* (that she will bring shame on her parents) and *personalization* (the idea that she is personally responsible for her parents' emotional well-being on top of their impoverished state, which she believes she has caused by siphoning money from the family coffers for her higher education). Finally, she engages in *"should" statements*, berating herself with thoughts that she must do better in the future and flagellating herself with the imagined consequences of failing to do so. See if you can take each of Janet's cognitive distortions and act as her CBT therapist, finding the questions that will help lead her to less morbid conclusions and improve her mood. Then skip to Table 6 and look at some of the questions that a skillful CBT therapist might ask her.

TABLE 6. Questions That a Skillful CBT Therapist Might Ask Janet

- "What is the evidence that your professor despises you?"
- "What have your past interactions with this professor been like?"
- "What kind of feedback did he give you on this paper?"
- "What about on other assignments?"
- "How do you think the professor regards the students who got an A on this assignment?"
- "What about the students who got a C . . . or an F?"

[These questions are geared toward disputing mind reading and black-or-white thinking based on empirical evidence.]

- "What written or verbal feedback have you received on your past performance from professors in other courses?"

[Look for evidence that some professors hold her in high regard.]

- "Let's assume this one professor truly thinks you are a dunce. So what? Could you live with that? How would you regard a professor who forms judgments of students on the basis of a single paper grade?"
- "What is the evidence that a B is a poor grade on this particular paper? What was the class average and the grade distribution?"
- "What does this single B mean for your overall grade in this particular course?"
- "How much is your final grade determined by this paper?"
- "How are you doing in the other areas that will factor into your grade?"

[If possible, mathematically work out what it would take to earn an A through an F and the estimated likelihood of each outcome.]

- "What would it mean to you if you ended up with an A, B, C . . . F in this course?"

[This explores and challenges the personal significance of this course in Janet's life. Once again, it confronts her all-or-nothing thinking, showing her that there are degrees of excellence and keeping her away from gravitating toward the extremes.]

- "How would your cumulative GPA or overall academic standing be affected?"
- "What is the evidence that your parents are actually ashamed of you?"
- "What have they said to you about your academic performance?"
- "You say that your parents have made sacrifices to send you to school. What would they say if they were here now?"

(cont.)

TABLE 6 (*cont.*)

[The degree of sacrifice involved may not be as great as Janet makes it out to be, and they may be happy to do it.]

- "What do your parents actually expect from you in return for their financial support?" [It's probably not straight As.]
- "Given this grade, what is the worst thing you can imagine happening in terms of your academic performance?"
- "What is the best thing that could happen?"
- "What is the likelihood of each outcome, from 0 to 100?"
- "What is actually the most realistic outcome?"

[You may recognize we used the same favorite techniques for Jack. They are widely applicable and extremely helpful.]

- "What makes for a successful and fulfilling life?"
- "What other ways do you have for measuring success in your life?"
- "How much does your performance in this course realistically contribute to future successes in each of these important areas?"

Identifying Your Core Negative Beliefs

Once you begin to log your negative thoughts regularly, you may find that they cluster around certain themes that come up again and again, sometimes with maddening regularity, especially during your depressions. These themes or patterns are called *core beliefs*, and they often seem to drive the negative thoughts. Melissa, the public relations specialist discussed earlier, believed that unless she chose a career path that pleased her parents, she would not be living a valuable and worthwhile life. That was a core belief, which filled her with self-doubts and made her very unhappy. Although the therapy she received was not strictly CBT, identifying that core belief and correcting it proved key to her recovery.

Peggy, another person with SAD whom I treated, had a core belief that she was stupid and incompetent, based no doubt on messages she had received as a child. Even though she had tested very well in school and had all sorts of academic laurels to her credit, whenever winter rolled around, she would feel like the dunce of the class. At those times she believed she was a fraud and teachers had given her good grades because they liked her, not because she had earned them.

Although Peggy's feelings of incompetence were no doubt fueled in part by the concentration difficulties so common in winter depressions, her repeated tendency to minimize her accomplishments and generalize her winter difficulties to encompass her entire life reached the level of a core belief.

Some core beliefs, like Peggy's, revolve around your concept of yourself: for example, a belief that you are defective, inadequate, vulnerable, or a failure. Other core beliefs pertain to your view of the world: for example, that you will be abandoned or disliked, or that you will or should be punished. Just as it can be very helpful to challenge your distorted cognitive thinking, it is useful to challenge your core beliefs, which is the next step in this program.

As you can see, a trained CBT therapist will energetically press the patient to challenge her ANTs and, in doing so, help the patient challenge them on her own. It is not quick or easy—but neither is straightening out your golf swing or your bridge game. Both Janet and Jack could benefit from extensive CBT work. On reading their brief vignettes, Kelly Rohan commented, "Both could take sessions of hammering away at the ANTs to make progress, and both are screaming of underlying core beliefs that complicate things. For Jack it's 'I'm unlovable and unattractive,' while for Janet it's 'I'm incompetent and I must be perfect.'"

Challenging Your Core Negative Beliefs

You might already be able to guess the elements of this next step. Log your core beliefs, dispute them, and, as always, practice this activity regularly. Judith Beck, director of the Beck Institute for Cognitive Behavior Therapy, has constructed the Core Belief Worksheet, which is very useful for this task (see Appendix B). Here's how you can use the worksheet. On the top of the sheet, write down the core belief that you wish to change. For example, Janet, the student who obtained a B+ grade on her paper, might jot down "I am inadequate and will never amount to anything." Assign a percentage to the most and the least that you ever hold the core belief, for example, 80% and 40%, respectively. On the left-hand side of the page, write those points of evidence that support your core belief; on the right, write those points that are against the belief. Follow each negative statement with a "BUT" and a rebuttal. For example, Janet might jot down "I earned a B on a paper in a very important course" but might immediately follow that with "BUT it could have been a lot worse" or "BUT many people would be pleased with that grade." Then, on the right-hand side of the vertical line she would list evidence against her core belief, for example, "I have maintained an A average all semester." After sorting out the pros and cons very thoroughly, the next task is to come up with a new, more realistic core belief, which would be written on the bottom of the paper. In Janet's case that might be "I'm a good student with a very promising future, and though I'm not always perfect, nobody is." Then ask yourself "How much do I believe this new core belief?" and "How much do I believe the original core belief?" Assign percentages to answer these two questions and see how the new percentages compare with the initial ones. Feel free to make extra copies of the form as needed.

Maintaining Gains and Preventing Relapse

As I mentioned, those people with SAD in Rohan's study who had been treated with CBT the previous year were less likely to relapse the following winter than those treated with light therapy alone. Studies of people with nonseasonal forms of depression have also found that both cognitive and behavioral techniques can help prevent relapse. So, watch out for the return of the ANTs and be ready to exterminate them at first sight, using the techniques outlined in this chapter. Likewise, guard against the tendency to retreat from enjoyable activities. For those seeking more information about CBT for SAD, I highly recommend Rohan's book, *Coping with the Seasons*, which is listed in the Resources section.

Other Forms of Therapy

Most skillful therapists combine different forms of therapy to achieve the best results. "Insight-oriented therapy" refers to a process of exploring the basis of various symptoms as a way of providing the patient with understanding and relief. For example, one woman with SAD who was in her mid-40s went into psychotherapy to help resolve the guilt she felt at having been the only healthy child out of six siblings. A middle-aged man with SAD struggled for years on his PhD thesis but was unable to complete it, not because of any intellectual limitation but because it raised anxiety in him about competing with his father, who had been much less successful than he was.

Other forms of therapy have been developed to deal with the long-term consequences of traumas, which can arise from a wide variety of situations such as combat stress, rape, or child sexual abuse. The scope of these various therapies goes beyond the present book.

In Chapter 11, I discuss two different forms of meditation that might hold some promise as potential treatments for depression: Transcendental Meditation (TM) and mindfulness-based cognitive therapy (MBCT).

Finally, it is important to remember that the family often plays a key role in the well-being of the individual—so some form of family therapy may be valuable at times.

Like all effective treatments, however, psychotherapy is not without hazards. Probing a person's past and stirring up buried secrets, while very helpful in some cases, is not universally so. Psychotherapy can sometimes amplify feelings of depression and anxiety and should be performed only by a skilled and properly trained therapist. That person should also be familiar with the biological treatments of depression so that the patient is not allowed to spin his or her wheels discussing childhood conflicts while an ongoing depression goes untreated.

Choosing a Psychotherapist

It is important to choose your therapist carefully. It is surprising to think that the same person who might take several days researching a car purchase—consulting *Consumer Reports* and friends, visiting several dealerships, and test-driving cars—might head straight for the Yellow Pages to find a therapist. A therapist is someone with whom you need to be able to share your most important personal thoughts and feelings. That person's judgment, training, and suitability for *you* should be the primary basis for your choice. How do you find such a person?

Recommendations from other professionals are often a good guide, as are recommendations from people currently in treatment with a trusted professional. Start with a health professional—or friend—

whom you respect. Briefly explain to this person the type of problem you are dealing with. Then ask his or her opinion as to who might be suitable for you. If possible, ask more than one professional (or friend), to see whether the same name appears on more than one list. Once you have obtained one or two names, set up an appointment to interview the prospective therapist.

A therapist you are interviewing should, of course, ask you questions about your problem. Consider whether the questions are on target:

- Does the therapist appear to be exploring the problem thoroughly, asking about it from different angles?

- Does he or she seem to understand what you are saying—not just intellectually but also emotionally?

- Does he or she appear empathic—on the same wavelength as you?

These early impressions are important and should be taken into consideration in making your decision.

Remember, although medical doctors, psychologists, and social workers may all be able to provide psychotherapy, only medical doctors can prescribe antidepressant medications. If you need both medications and psychotherapy, it is possible to obtain both types of help from a psychiatrist or to obtain medications from a doctor and therapy from someone else. I have worked with patients in both of these formats, and either situation can be successful. If two professionals are involved, both should be competent, and they should work well as a team. The patient's responsibility is to keep each professional informed in general terms of what the other is doing.

You are certainly entitled to ask questions of the prospective therapist. What is his or her background and training? Does he or she subscribe to any particular school of therapy? If these questions are asked in an ordinary, matter-of-fact manner, they should be met with ordinary, matter-of-fact replies. Any defensiveness about the replies, questions in response to your questions (such as "Why do you want to know?"), or interpretations (such as "It seems as though you suspect my competency") might reasonably raise suspicion about insecurity on the part of the therapist.

At the end of the initial consultation, the therapist should provide a formulation of the problem—a diagnosis and some clarification of the issues—as well as specific recommendations about treatment. Sometimes, however, if the situation appears to be complicated, more than one meeting might be necessary before the therapist is ready to provide a formulation and recommendations. It's important for you to consider this formulation and these recommendations as just *one* way to see the problem. There may be other ways to see it as well, and you may wish to seek other opinions before making up your mind about which therapist is right for you.

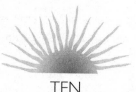

TEN

Antidepressant Medications

> ♦ How much is it reasonable to expect from these medications?
>
> ♦ What are their side effects and liabilities?
>
> ♦ What are the differences among available antidepressants?
>
> ♦ What is the best choice for you?
>
> ♦ How do these drugs work?
>
> By now it is common wisdom that antidepressant medications have revolutionized the treatment of depression. In this chapter I will present the evidence for the value of antidepressants in treating SAD. The questions above are particularly important because light therapy is not right for everybody. Some people do not respond to light therapy, many respond only partially, and others find it too cumbersome or inconvenient.

To date, dozens of studies have been undertaken to examine the value of medications in the treatment of SAD. Although the sample sizes in these studies were small, the results were basically positive. There is every reason to expect that antidepressants *would* work for SAD since it is a form of depression—and they do.

One particularly interesting set of studies, which I conducted with Jack Modell, who was at the pharmaceutical company GlaxoSmith-Kline at the time, explored the possibility of starting antidepressant usage in people with SAD in the autumn before the onset of symptoms. We studied a long-acting form of the antidepressant Wellbutrin (bupropion) in more than 1,000 people with SAD and found that the antidepressant reduced the risk of developing an episode of SAD the following winter by almost 50%. Most people tolerated the drug well, and side effects were modest. The only side effects that were present to a meaningful degree were dry mouth, nausea, constipation, flatulence, and weight loss. To my knowledge, these are the first studies to show that depression can be prevented by starting an antidepressant before it begins. In June 2006 the FDA approved Wellbutrin XL for preventing episodes of winter depression in people with a history of severe SAD.

Another interesting finding to emerge from the Wellbutrin XL prevention study was that patients did not relapse after the medication was discontinued at the beginning of spring. This demonstrates that people with SAD often need to be treated only during the fall and winter months, when they are at particular risk. Their antidepressant medications can often be tapered or even discontinued toward the end of winter. Curiously, sometimes medications that are well tolerated in the winter begin to cause side effects when spring arrives, probably because the brain's chemistry is changing with the change of seasons. This often is a signal that it is time to reduce medication dosage. On the other hand, some people with SAD may need continued medications throughout the year.

Arlene, a 45-year-old financial advisor, was one of my patients who participated in the clinical trial. I had diagnosed her as suffering from SAD some 3 years earlier and had treated her with light therapy. It worked, but she hated it. The light box offended her aesthetic sensibilities and served as a constant unwelcome reminder to her that there was something "wrong" with her. The dawn simulator woke her husband, which he found unacceptable. She was thrilled at the prospect of an alternative. For Arlene, Wellbutrin XL turned out to work just as well as light therapy with no ill effects, and she has now used it happily for the past two winters, starting it in the fall and stopping it in the spring.

While some people may want to prevent the symptoms of SAD

before they start, others may prefer to wait for symptoms to develop before initiating treatment. Arlene clearly fell into the first group and was unwilling to suffer even the beginning of her winter doldrums before starting treatment. But evidence suggests that antidepressant treatment will be effective even if initiated after symptoms begin.

Although most evidence regarding the use of antidepressants for SAD comes from the Wellbutrin studies, there is every reason to believe—based on clinical experience and our knowledge of how anti-depressants work—that other antidepressants will also be effective. Ideally they should be prescribed by a psychiatrist who has both skill with medications and knowledge of SAD. In practice, however, pri-mary care physicians might be able to manage as well for many people. Regardless of discipline, it is very important to find a knowledgeable and empathic physician to ensure that you get good care.

Finding the right antidepressant or combination of antidepres-sants is a matter of trial and error. A skilled clinician knows that and keeps trying until the best fit is found. Although many people with SAD respond to a variety of different antidepressants, some do not. For example, I treated one man with many different antidepressants until I hit on one that worked—in this instance, Cymbalta (duloxetine). For someone else, another antidepressant might be the magic bullet.

Common Concerns and Considerations about Taking Antidepressants

All sorts of reasonable concerns arise about taking antidepressant med-ications:

- Will the drugs harm you?
- Will you feel too good and get hooked on them?
- If you feel better, will it be the result of the pills or your own efforts?
- You may always have been told to examine the roots of your problems and solve them from the ground up. Now someone is telling you not to worry about roots and origins. Just take the pills and you'll feel better. Can it be so simple?

Many people are afraid that, instead of alleviating their symptoms, an antidepressant will change them for the worse. This rarely happens. Rather, most people feel that the antidepressant allows them to be their best self. In the minority who experience unwelcome changes, the antidepressant can simply be changed or withdrawn.

The thought of taking a mood-altering drug may, however, trigger associations with dependence or addiction. Let me assure you that antidepressant drugs do not generally cause an immediate high, nor are they addictive, though they should not generally be stopped abruptly as this can result in unpleasant discontinuation symptoms (see pp. 218 and 221).

Antidepressants generally don't make people "high," are not addictive, and are not "just an easy way out."

Some people may feel that taking an antidepressant is the easy way out, an evasion of responsibility for uncovering the cause of a problem and rooting it out. This idea can actually be harmful, as it readily triggers thoughts that you are somehow to blame for the depression and responsible for fixing it yourself. This way of thinking plays into the guilt that so often bedevils those afflicted by depression and runs counter to the modern understanding that clinical depression is an illness involving disturbed brain biochemistry.

One reason it may be difficult to accept the medical model of depression is that there is no good laboratory test for it. We have to depend on a person's history for diagnosis, which in the case of SAD is much easier to make than in other depressions, both because of the seasonal recurrences and the reactivity to changes in environmental light. Invest some time and energy in finding a good doctor who will take your SAD symptoms seriously and knows his or her medications. Consult with your doctor about which medication will be best for you, using the rest of this chapter as a guide in this discussion.

Many people are concerned about how long they will have to remain on medications. This is easier to predict for people with SAD than for those with other forms of depression because SAD is usually a self-limiting condition. When summer comes, symptoms generally resolve. In some cases, however, medications may be helpful even in the summertime. Another concern that I have heard from time to time is a fear that antidepressant medications will cause some permanent change or damage. Fortunately, chronic side effects are rare, and there is no evidence whatsoever that any long-term damage to the brain occurs. In fact, some studies suggest that long-term antidepressant use may actually protect brain cells against the damage that can occur as a result of chronic untreated depression.

Side Effects of Medications

Concerns about side effects are common and valid. People vary greatly in their tendency to develop side effects. On one end of the spectrum is the individual who develops none at all; on the other end is the person who develops many side effects from a host of different antidepressants at dosages so low that no beneficial effects are possible. Because of this wide variability, many psychiatrists choose to start with low dosages of the medication of choice and build up after seeing how well a person tolerates it.

The side effects of antidepressant medications differ from drug to drug and are discussed at greater length under each specific heading. For many antidepressants, common side effects include sedation, weight gain, dizziness, sexual difficulties, and a cluster of symptoms known as "anticholinergic side effects"—such as constipation, dry mouth, urinary retention, and blurred vision. Table 7 lists some of the most commonly used antidepressants, along with their suspected mechanisms of action and common side effects.

Rarely, in the first week or two of starting an antidepressant, people can feel worse—for example, activated, agitated, or even suicidal. Be sure to tell your doctor should these unusual symptoms develop so that appropriate remedial actions can be taken.

Remember that sudden discontinuation of most antidepressants can have unpleasant effects, including abnormal dreams, "pins and needles," dizziness, mood changes, irritability, strange sensations, and recurrence of depression, to name just a few of many possible symptoms. For some antidepressants, those that leave the system quickly, this may be more of a problem than for others. I suggest that you discuss the question of discontinuation with your

> *When it is desirable to stop an antidepressant, it should be tapered, wherever possible.*

TABLE 7. Brief Overview of Antidepressants

Brand (generic) name	Neurotransmitters affected	Potential advantages	Potential disadvantages
Wellbutrin (bupropion)	DA +++ NE ++	Less likely to cause sexual difficulties and weight gain. Can prevent depression if started early in season.	Not as good for anxiety; may increase risk of seizures in vulnerable individuals.
Selective serotonin reuptake inhibitors (SSRIs)			
Prozac (fluoxetine)	SE +++	All are effective. Approved for some anxiety disorders as well as depression.	Side effects: Problems with sexual functioning, lethargy, weight gain.
Zoloft (sertraline)	SE +++		
Paxil (paroxetine)	SE +++		
Celexa (citalopram)	SE +++		
Luvox (fluvoxamine)	SE +++		
Viibryd (vilazodone)	SE +++		
Serotonin and norepinephrine reuptake inhibitors (SNRIs)			
Effexor (venlafaxine)	SE ++ NE ++	Approved for treatment of some anxiety disorders as well as depression.	Can cause increased blood pressure and some SSRI-type side effects.

(cont.)

TABLE 7 (cont.)

Brand (generic) name	Neurotransmitters affected	Potential advantages	Potential disadvantages
Cymbalta (duloxetine)	SE + NE +++	May be helpful when there is pain as well as depression.	Can cause nausea, dry mouth, drowsiness, constipation, and insomnia.
Savella (milnacipran)*	SE + NE +++		

Tricyclic antidepressants (TCAs)

Tofranil (imipramine)	SE ++ NE ++	All tricyclics are effective and may help anxiety as well as depression. Their sleep-inducing side effects can initially be an advantage for those with insomnia.	Tricyclics often have more side effects than modern antidepressants. These include dry mouth, constipation, blurred vision, fatigue, and weight gain. Dangerous in overdose.
Anafranil (chlorimipramine)	SE +++ NE +		
Elavil (amitriptyline)	SE ++ NE ++		
Norpramin (desipramine)	NE +++ SE +		
Pamelor/Aventyl (nortriptyline)	SE ++ NE ++		

Note. SE = serotonin; NE = norepinephrine; DA = dopamine; + = slight; ++ = moderate; +++ = marked.

*At the time of printing this medication was approved for fibromyalgia but not depression in the United States; elsewhere it is approved for both.

doctor ahead of time. Also, be sure not to stop your antidepressants abruptly without consulting your doctor first.

The Pros and Cons of Using Antidepressant Medications

A cost–benefit analysis should certainly be undertaken every time medications are used. What good is this medication likely to do? What harm might result? In the case of antidepressant medications, this analysis should be a shared process between you and your doctor, perhaps to an even greater degree than for other forms of medicine. That's because many of the symptoms of depression—such as sadness, guilt, and feelings of low self-worth—are known only to you. The same applies for side effects. Your psychiatrist will depend largely on *your* evaluation of how bad both symptoms and side effects are. In addition, since you have to live with both the symptoms of the illness and the side effects of the medicine, it seems only fair that you should have the major say in whether to be on the medications or not and which one to choose.

So where does the psychiatrist fit into the picture? Your psychiatrist should educate you about the nature of the illness, the available treatment options, and their potential benefits and possible risks. You should be informed about the psychiatrist's experience with both the drug and the illness and how it pertains to your particular situation. Although the psychiatrist cannot know for sure how a drug will work in any particular case, you should understand why he or she is recommending a certain drug over others at a particular time. You should be given an idea as to what effects—both good and bad—the drug might have and when these effects are likely to occur. In addition, the psychiatrist should explain where the medication fits into the overall game plan for the treatment of your problems and what other steps will be taken if it does not work well enough. You, in turn, should feel free to share your concerns about the medication, which may be influenced by earlier medication experiences. Ideally the doctor and patient should discuss the pros and cons of the medication together, and through such a dialogue the best decision is likely to be made.

Although most medications *can* cause a wide array of side effects, many of these are extremely unusual. In my own practice, I tend to discuss the most common side effects of a particular medication and note that other side effects may occur. I also recommend that my patients ask their pharmacist for the medication package insert, which they may or may not choose to read, but which is useful to have if any questions arise. If while on medications you develop any physical or psychological changes that have not been discussed fully, or about which you feel concerned, don't hesitate to contact your psychiatrist by phone rather than wait for the next visit.

In general, cost–benefit analysis greatly favors the use of antidepressant medications, especially when depression is moderate to severe, the individual is relatively healthy, and nonmedical alternatives (such as light therapy) seem unlikely to do the job by themselves. In addition, people with seasonal depressions seem to respond well to medications, and *I cannot think of one patient with SAD who could not be helped to some degree by a combination of light, antidepressant medication, and the other strategies outlined in this book. Despite the benefits of antidepressants, if symptoms can be treated successfully without medications, this course is often preferable.*

Medications Commonly Used in SAD

The discussion in this section is intended to inform you about some of the most useful medications available for the treatment of SAD in particular and depression in general so that you can participate in your doctor's recommended antidepressant treatment regimen in a more informed way. It should not, however, be construed as medical advice, which can be given only by a doctor.

Many different types of medications are available for treating depression (see Table 7). The choice of which drug to use first is an educated guess, based on the available literature, the nature of your problem, and the therapeutic and side-effect profile of the medication. I usually start either with Wellbutrin (bupropion) or a member of the selective serotonin reuptake inhibitor (SSRI) family such as Zoloft (sertraline) or Celexa (citalopram). If that doesn't work, then I will either shift to Cymbalta (duloxetine) or Effexor (venlafaxine) or try some combination of medications.

Because there is no scientific method at this time for reliably predicting the best antidepressants for a particular person, treatment often proceeds by trial and error. If the first choice doesn't work, the next should be tried. Sometimes you have to try several different drugs before you finally hit on the right one. It's a bit like having a large bunch of keys and trying each in turn until you find the one that turns a lock. But once the lock turns, the door opens, and new vistas appear. So it is for the depressed person who finally feels better and is able to enjoy life once again. It may be helpful to bear this image in mind if the first or second antidepressant fails to deliver its promised effect; otherwise, it is easy to become discouraged and give up prematurely when the next key on the bunch may be the right one.

All antidepressants take time to work. At least 3 weeks should be allowed after the medication has been administered *in sufficient dosage* before making a judgment about its effectiveness. Because of the wide variation in susceptibility to side effects, psychiatrists often choose to start a medication at a low dose and increase gradually. The only problem with this approach is that it will take longer for the medicine to have its full effect, so if you are severely depressed it may make sense for your doctor to start you on a higher dose and increase more rapidly. In people with SAD, antidepressant medications may be used either instead of light therapy or to supplement it. Light therapy may be only partially effective; an antidepressant may finish off the job. Also, if light therapy is used together with antidepressants, it is often possible to get by with smaller doses and fewer side effects. It is often necessary to adjust the dosage with the changing seasons—increasing it as the days become shorter and darker and decreasing it as the days become longer and brighter.

The ABCs of Neurotransmitters

The human brain consists of billions of neurons that communicate with each other at junctions known as "synapses." At the synapse an electrical message passing along the transmitting neuron causes the release of chemical messengers known as "neurotransmitters" that drift across the space between two neurons and stimulate special receptors on the receiving neuron. This transmits the electrical signal that continues to pass along the neural circuit. So it is that these amazing molecules, "neurotransmitters," drive the circuits that are responsible for every function mediated by the human brain, including the regulation of our moods. Once released, the neurotransmitters are taken back into the transmitting neuron (a process called "reuptake"), where they are broken down. Most of our antidepressants work by inhibiting the reuptake of these neurotransmitters, three of which have come under the most prominent scrutiny—serotonin, norepinephrine, and dopamine. A major difference between available antidepressants is their signature pattern of influence on the various neurotransmitters.

Brain neurotransmitter systems govern too many functions to cover in this simple introduction, so I'll mention just a few:

- Serotonin is important for inducing a calm, good mood and helping to restrain impulses such as displays of bad temper.
- Dopamine is important for reward pathways, pleasure, attention, and motivation.
- Norepinephrine increases alertness and energizes.

Now that you understand the symptoms of SAD, you can see why all these neurotransmitters might be important in its treatment. Table 7 shows how different available antidepressants affect different neurotransmitters. A few of these antidepressants are described below in greater detail.

Wellbutrin (Bupropion)

This drug is thought to work by influencing dopamine and norepinephrine. It comes in three different forms: immediate release (IR), sustained release (SR), and once-a-day extended release (XL). All three are available in generic form. The large SAD prevention study mentioned earlier in this chapter used the XL form of the drug.

Advantages of bupropion are that it is energizing and not associated with weight gain, sexual side effects, lethargy, or sedation. Bupropion may be particularly helpful when lethargy and sluggishness are a prominent part of the picture. Side effects in the SAD studies included dry mouth, nausea, constipation, flatulence, and weight loss, which occurred in a small proportion of people taking the drug. A rare but disturbing side effect is the occurrence of seizures. Therefore, people with a history of seizures would be advised to avoid this drug.

Selective Serotonin Reuptake Inhibitors (SSRIs)

As their name implies, these antidepressants work by selectively inhibiting the reuptake of serotonin. They are extremely popular for treating depression in general. Evidence suggests that they are also effective for treating winter depressions in those with SAD. There is no evidence that one of these is superior to any other in general, although in particular individuals one may prove to be better than others. Several of these are now available in generic form. They are particularly good when anxiety is a prominent part of the picture. Advantages include a low level of the type of side effects that bedeviled earlier antidepressants, such as constipation and dry mouth. Disadvantages include sexual side effects, fatigue, a sense of flattened emotions, and weight gain. These affect only some people taking these drugs, whereas others are lucky and experience no side effects at all. Sexual side effects may include decreased desire and greater difficulties with arousal and achieving orgasm.

SSRIs

Prozac (fluoxetine)

Zoloft (sertraline)

Paxil (paroxetine)

Luvox (fluvoxamine)

Celexa (citalopram)

Lexapro (escitalopram)

Viibryd (vilazodone)

Combined Serotonin and Norepinephrine Reuptake Inhibitors (SNRIs)

These drugs influence both serotonin and norepinephrine transmission. Effexor is available in both immediate and extended release (XR) preparations. Effexor has been approved for some anxiety disorders as well as for depression. Cymbalta works more powerfully on norepinephrine than on serotonin reuptake—so it is not interchangeable with Effexor. For

SNRIs

Effexor (venlafaxine)

Cymbalta (duloxetine)

example, Cymbalta is more helpful than Effexor in treating pain that may be associated with depression. Common side effects of Effexor include edginess, sedation, increased blood pressure, sleep disruption, and sexual side effects. Common side effects of Cymbalta include nausea, dry mouth, drowsiness, constipation, high blood pressure, and insomnia. In addition, Cymbalta might be harmful to the liver in those who drink excessively.

Tricyclic Antidepressants (TCAs)

These old workhorses date all the way back to the 1950s and for years were almost the only antidepressants available. They were superseded by the SSRIs and other modern drugs because they had many troublesome side effects such as dry mouth, constipation, blurred vision, seizures, and slowed-down conduction of electrical signals in the heart. If taken in overdose, they are far more dangerous than more modern drugs, and such overdoses can be fatal. Despite these problems, they remain useful drugs when newer ones are unable to do the job for one reason or another. In practice, though, I rarely use these medications for people with SAD.

TCAs

Norpramin (desipramine)

Tofranil (imipramine)

Pamelor (nortriptyline)

Elavil (amitriptyline)

Newer Antidepressants

Several newer antidepressants are wending their way down the pike as I update this book. Viibryd (vilazodone), which has been approved as an antidepressant on the U.S. market, works predominantly on serotonin systems. Savella (milnacipran), which has been approved in the United States for fibromyalgia but not yet as an antidepressant, works on both norepinephrine and serotonin systems. Finally, a novel antidepressant, Valdoxan (agomelatine), approved elsewhere but not yet in the United States, acts on melatonin receptors, as well as on serotonin receptors.

As yet, we have no data on how helpful these medications will be for SAD. Also, as of the time of writing, our experience with these drugs for depression in general is quite limited.

Combining Antidepressants with Light Therapy

In clinical practice, combining medications and light therapy is often more effective than either treatment alone and also may make it possible to get by with a lower medication dosage and less time in front of the lights. A potential disadvantage is that the treatments may compound each other's side effects. For example, a person may be more likely to experience hypomanic symptoms on a combination of light therapy and medications than on either treatment alone.

Sara's Story: Throwing the Kitchen Sink at It

Every now and then I encounter a person with SAD whose symptoms are either so severe or so resistant to simple remedies that every measure has to be taken to overcome them. You have to throw the kitchen sink at the problem. Sara was such a person.

Sara was a psychiatric nurse in her late 30s, married and without children, who lived and worked in rural Massachusetts. She had suffered from problems with the winter since she was 17 years old and had been treated for them with psychotherapy and numerous medications, which helped to only a small degree.

Life became much more difficult for Sara in the 2 years before she consulted me, starting with a serious depression that occurred, quite uncharacteristically, during the summer shortly after she quit smoking. The unusual reason for this was that nurses who smoked would get the chance to take patients who were smokers outside into the sunshine for frequent smoke breaks. Nonsmokers like Sara, on the other hand, were required to remain indoors on a dark psychiatric ward for long hours and had little access to bright natural light. Sara remained depressed through the summer, into the next fall and winter, and was still depressed when I saw her at the end of the second summer.

What followed was an extensive series of interventions to help free Sara of her depressions. Light therapy (plus dawn simulation) and antidepressants at maximum dosages were of little benefit. Only trips to Florida and Mexico seemed to move her spirits in the right direction.

Luckily her husband was extremely supportive, and together they crafted a plan. Sara would make several brief trips to Florida as a "safety net" for the forthcoming winter when the depression became too bad. Not only did this strategy prove valuable, but just knowing that the plan was in place was a great comfort.

Sara began to feel depressed again in early August, and I started to treat her with a combination of light therapy (1 to 2 hours per day) and antidepressants, in escalating dosage. She exercised regularly and used a dawn simulator in an attempt to hold the time of dawn constant as the days became shorter. Unfortunately, despite the combination of light, medications, and therapy, depression returned and began its inexorable downhill course.

She used her planned time away to good effect, and the three 1-week vacations, scheduled for December, January, and February, all significantly lifted her spirits. She was able to tell her husband just how bad she felt at times during the winter, and he began to appreciate their need to make major lifestyle changes to accommodate her problem. Relocation seemed like the only viable option, and together they chose a community in Florida, to which they relocated. Since Sara has lived in Florida, her moods have been considerably better, and she has never expressed a word of regret about her choice to leave her home, family, and friends for sunnier climes.

I have deliberately included a story of someone who has found neither a quick nor an easy path to recovery. There are, of course, many others who, like Sara, have needed to combine multiple types of treatment, including relocation, to conquer their winter depressions. Despite these efforts and sacrifices, or rather because of them, almost everybody can resolve the problem of winter depression one way or another. The message of Sara's story for those of you out there whose path to recovery has also been difficult is "Don't despair." There are all kinds of things that can help, either individually or in combination, and I recommend that you try different approaches at the advice and under the supervision of a good professional. Keep well informed and up to date on the latest research developments. Even if you don't completely overcome your SAD symptoms this winter, who knows what new discoveries next winter will bring?

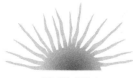

ELEVEN

Meditation for SAD

I want to go soon and live away by the pond where I shall
hear only the wind whispering among the reeds—It will
be a success if I shall have left myself behind. But my
friends ask what I will do when I get there? Will it not be
employment enough to watch the progress of the seasons?
—HENRY DAVID THOREAU

 ● With research evidence showing that depression (and anxiety)
can be eased by meditation, could meditation help you with
SAD?

 ● Would you consider spending about 20 minutes once or twice
a day to reap additional improvements in your SAD symptoms?

 ● How does meditation affect brain waves, hormones, blood
pressure, and other physiological processes in a way that may
help SAD sufferers?

 ● What might different forms of meditation have to offer you?

While we are still lacking controlled studies exploring the effects
of specific types of meditation on SAD, there is mounting clinical
and anecdotal evidence that transcendental meditation, mindfulness meditation, and loving-kindness compassion may ease the
symptoms of SAD in the same way that research has shown
them to improve depression, anxiety, and stress.

*A*s we have seen, winter means different things to different people. But for many creatures living at a distance from the equator, it offers an invitation (or sends a directive) to withdraw from the world—even perhaps briefly. Despite the round of parties that enliven the holiday season, an attempt perhaps to defy this natural trend, there persists a general sense of shutting down. Schools and businesses close. People retreat into their houses; bears into their caves; Thoreau to his shack by Walden Pond. With less to do outdoors, the season seems perfectly suited to retreating within the self—for observation, contemplation and, indeed, meditation.

This concept—a connection between winter and meditation—has long been of theoretical interest to me. In recent years, however, it has taken a practical turn as I myself have personally experienced tremendous benefits from meditation year round, but more so in the winter—a particularly stressful time for me as it is for all people with SAD.

How I began to meditate is a story in itself—one that strangely parallels how I stumbled onto SAD and light therapy. Once again, a patient provided the first clue and encouraged me to set out on a journey of exploration. Just as Herb Kern led the way for me and my colleagues to pursue seasonal changes in mood and behavior, so this more recent patient, a young student named Paul, first suggested to me the possibility that meditation might hold promise as a powerful remedy for various emotional disorders. I realized, of course—though I greatly underestimated its powers—that meditation might help a broad spectrum of people relax and feel less stressed. What was quite novel to me, despite over three decades as a researcher and practicing psychiatrist, was that meditation was powerful enough to soothe the nerves even of highly stressed and anxious people, as well as to enliven those who felt depleted and downcast as a result of too much stress, too little resilience, or both.

Paul suffered from bipolar disorder and, by the time we met, had already been through several devastating rounds of mania and depression. We managed to bring these under control with the help of a powerful cocktail of mood stabilizers, but stability did not in itself bring happiness. He felt that something was missing. At that time Paul met another person with bipolar disorder whose story echoed his own. This other person recommended that Paul regularly practice Transcendental Meditation (TM), a skill he had learned previously but had only dabbled in halfheartedly. Paul followed this advice and, true to his friend's promise, began to feel "truly happy 90% of the time."

Of special interest to us here is the seasonality of Paul's moods and his extreme sensitivity to environmental light, which was so marked that during the summer he had to use blackout shades in his bedroom to prevent being awakened by the first rays of dawn. Likewise, he had to remain in dim indoor lighting in the evening to prevent the development of insomnia and mania—despite taking multiple mood-stabilizing medications. Conversely, in winter, he would experience many of the SAD symptoms we have already encountered, especially low energy, a downbeat mood, and—most painful to this aspiring filmmaker—lack of creativity.

Paul's regular TM practice not only helped stabilize his mood swings, but by destressing him, gave him more energy and zest in the winter. In addition, meditation helped Paul focus and get things done—no small feat for this young man who, along with his bipolar disorder, had a lifelong history of ADHD and organizational difficulties. I told Paul that I had learned TM as a medical student but had let it lapse. He encouraged me to have my technique refreshed—which I did—and to practice regularly. The results were astonishing. I became calmer and more likely to respond thoughtfully than react reflexively to stresses and challenges. So pleased was I with the effects of TM on Paul and myself that I began to recommend it to others—with excellent results. I looked into the literature on TM and was so impressed with the large number of high-quality papers on the subject in peer-reviewed journals that I decided to write a book on the subject—*Transcendence: Healing and Transformation through Transcendental Meditation* (see Resources).

Of particular relevance here, I became less stressed during winter and had more energy for both enjoyable activities and the chores of everyday life. With Paul's observations and my own in mind, I set out to find other people with SAD who had benefited from meditation. To my surprise, this was easier than I had anticipated. I am excited to bring to your attention the latest news about this ancient practice: besides all its other benefits, meditation can also help people with SAD.

In this chapter, we will explore what two forms of meditation have to offer those who struggle through the winter. Although most Westerners know something about meditation, many lump together all the different types, which derive from many great cultures. That would be like lumping together all the different types of psychotherapy. Each type of meditation requires that the meditator perform a different task to achieve the desired effect, which may also differ from one form of meditation to another.

To put the different forms of meditation into perspective, researchers Fred Travis of Maharishi University of Management and Jonathan Shear of Virginia Commonwealth University suggested three broad categories. They classify TM into the category of *automatic self-transcending*. What they mean by this is that although a mantra or word-sound is initially used in a TM session, it tends to disappear during meditation—it transcends itself. The other two categories are *open monitoring* and *focused attention*.

Open monitoring, as its name suggests, involves nonjudgmental awareness of the moment-to-moment content of experience—for example, the breath, bodily sensations, thoughts, feelings, movements, and the environment. An attitude of openness, curiosity, and acceptance is encouraged. Focused attention, on the other hand, involves voluntary and sustained attention on a chosen object, for example, a candle flame, a mandala, or a beloved image. Examples of open monitoring meditation include Vipassana (insight) and Zen. Examples of focused attention include loving-kindness compassion. Mindfulness meditation, which we will consider in greater detail below, combines elements of both open monitoring and single-focus meditation.

Studies of electroencephalogram (EEG) patterns during meditation reveal different EEG changes during these different types of meditation, as one would expect. Given these differences, one form of meditation may work better for you than another. Therefore, if you try one form of meditation and it doesn't work for you, don't give up on the whole idea of meditation before trying a different type. Also, remember that many forms of treatment work only if you adhere to them regularly. Just as you won't get the full effect of light therapy or exercise unless you adhere to a

> If one form of meditation doesn't work for you, don't give up on the whole idea of meditation before trying another form. You need to practice meditation regularly for a while—say, a few months—before you have a good idea whether it is likely to benefit you or not.

regular schedule, so it is with meditation. And the downside of practicing any of these treatments in a desultory way is that you might easily conclude that they don't work, and thereby miss out on something that could turn out to be very valuable.

Transcendental Meditation

There is something beyond our mind which abides in silence within our mind. It is the supreme mystery beyond thought. Let one's mind . . . rest on that and not rest on anything else.
—*Maitri Upanishad*

TM was introduced to India and the West in the middle of the last century by Maharishi Mahesh Yogi, who took an ancient Vedic technique, distilled its essence, and adapted it so that it can be practiced easily in many different settings. Ideally, you should practice TM for 20 minutes twice a day, sitting comfortably with your eyes closed. The technique involves using a mantra, which is a word-sound, in a specific way that is taught by a qualified TM teacher on a one-on-one basis. Initial instruction has seven steps: two lectures and a personal interview with the teacher, followed by four teaching sessions on four consecutive days. Ideally, the fledgling meditator then follows up with the teacher, maybe weekly for the first month, then once a month until the technique has been clearly established.

The technique's name—"transcendental"—is based on a state of consciousness that its practice reliably induces. The key elements of this state are a sense of boundlessness with regard to time and space, an alertness without specific content, and a blissful sense of calm. TM practitioners refer to this state as "transcendence," which is described above in a quote from one of the Upanishads, an ancient Vedic text.

Physiological research has shown transcendence to be associated with certain changes in brain-wave patterns and hormonal secretion. Specifically the EEG shows increased alpha waves (a brain rhythm associated with a calm, relaxed state), especially in the frontal regions of the brain, which are important for judgment and decision making— so-called "executive functions." Of even greater interest, during transcendence alpha waves show more "coherence," a term that refers to the degree of correspondence between brain-wave patterns in different brain regions. Greater levels of coherence are associated with improved levels of effectiveness in sports and business. After a TM session, levels of the soothing hormone prolactin increase in the bloodstream. Levels of prolactin also increase in the bloodstream when people rest at night in the dark, as well as in nursing mothers and roosting chickens— all situations that call for a calm state of mind. In summary, there is physiological evidence that explains how the regular practice of TM may induce calmness and improve efficiency, just as its practitioners report.

As you may recall from Chapter 4, Tom Wehr and colleagues at the NIMH conducted some landmark experiments in which they asked people to lie in darkened rooms for two different durations of darkness: 14 versus 10 hours, corresponding roughly to the duration of darkness on a winter versus a summer night in the Washington, DC, area. The researchers compared the subjects' psychological, sleep, and physiological changes under those two conditions. They found that during the 14-hour nights people reported sleeping in two distinct blocks, separated by an interval of wakefulness lasting, on average, about 2 hours. During this interval of wakefulness, people reported feeling a sense of pleasant, calm alertness, along with a "crystal-clear consciousness." This description is highly reminiscent of the state of transcendence. Interestingly, during the 14-hour nights, blood levels of prolactin increased more than during the shorter nights—another change reminiscent of a state of transcendence.

For thousands of years before the widespread availability of bright indoor lighting—from Homer all the way up to modern times—writers described sleeping in a way that resembles the sleep patterns of Wehr's subjects during their long nights. Specifically, up until the early 20th century, people reported experiencing a "first sleep" and a "second sleep," separated by a period of wakefulness, which was known as "the watch." These descriptions are nicely documented in a book by A. R. Ekirch called *At Day's Close: Night in Times Past* (see Resources). I elaborate on these resemblances in my book *Transcendence*.

One reason people are so stressed nowadays may be that with the ubiquitous presence of bright indoor lighting, we have lost the practice of lying in bed for long periods and no longer enjoy the nightly psychological and physiological benefits of a state of calm attentiveness, coupled by pleasant feelings and crystal-clear consciousness. Perhaps one way that TM helps depressed and nondepressed people alike is by replacing something we used to enjoy during the winter nights of long ago that has been lost in our hectic modern lives.

To begin to understand how TM might help depression and other stress-related conditions, it is useful to understand how it reduces the effects of physical stress. This beneficial influence has been studied most extensively in relation to blood pressure—a common and potentially dangerous effect of stress on the body. A survey of nine random controlled studies shows that regularly practicing TM significantly reduces blood pressure. These findings have several important implications: First, reducing blood pressure would be expected to have major health benefits. It is not without reason that high blood pressure has been called "the silent killer." Second, since lowered blood pressure is found at varying times after the preceding TM session, the effects of TM appear to persist throughout the day. Finally, reduced blood pressure indicates reduced activity in that part of the nervous system known to be involved in responses to stress—the sympathetic nervous system. The reduction in blood pressure in people who practice TM regularly is almost certainly due to its stress-relieving effects. Let us consider each of these implications in turn.

As expected, TM's ability to decrease blood pressure does in fact pay off. The most dramatic evidence for this comes from two follow-up studies. The first, a retrospective investigation of the death records of people who had previously participated in controlled blood pressure studies (such as the studies mentioned in the previous paragraph) revealed that those assigned to the TM group went on to have a 23% reduction in overall mortality compared to those who had received health education lectures. This finding was all the more remarkable in that the investigators had had no contact with the research participants in the intervening years (7 years on average)—so nobody even knew whether people had continued to meditate. The second was a *prospective* study of about 200 people at risk for cardiac disease who were randomly assigned to TM or health education, along with their regular cardiac care, and then followed over time. After an average of 5 years the TM group had a 47% reduction in their risk of heart attack, stroke, or death from any cause. This is especially impressive when you consider that TM showed significant benefits over and above regular medical treatment.

The second implication—the carryover effects of TM throughout the day—is particularly relevant to the potential benefit for people with SAD. There is evidence both from personal reports and EEG studies that after practicing TM for a while people begin to experience transcendence and greater calmness outside of TM sessions, throughout the day. Over time, EEG tracings begin to show evidence of coherence even during the day when people are not meditating. Along with more enduring feelings of transcendence, people report an increased awareness of their surroundings, which they experience with greater vividness and in more fine-grained detail. This is often accompanied by a deeper sense of connection with other people and with the universe as a whole. You can imagine how the deepening of such pleasant feelings may have antidepressant effects.

Finally, anything that decreases stress is of interest to people with SAD, for whom even small challenges can feel highly stressful during the dark days of winter. There is substantial evidence that TM cushions the response to experimental stressors, such as loud noises, grisly movies, and painful stimuli. In reaction to the first two of these stressors, after showing an initial stress response, meditators settled down more rapidly than controls and did not exhibit the further "false alarm" responses that were seen in nonmeditators. In the pain study (involving sticking a finger into very hot water), meditators showed less marked brain responses than nonmeditators, as measured by imaging techniques, even though they rated their pain level as severely as the nonmeditators.

What all these studies suggest is that the regular practice of TM buffers people from the impact of all sorts of stresses that assail them on a daily basis—it improves their shock absorbers. Alex, an accountant who was in his early 30s when he entered a research study of the potential benefits of TM for people with bipolar disorder, found this to be the case. Here is what he had to say after 3 months of TM practice:

> Since the start of the study, since integrating TM into my daily routine, it has helped the spikes and valleys. Normally, if an intensely negative

event were to occur, I would be a mess for a week or longer. Now, when I have a similar, almost exact same trauma, I am out for only a day. So yes, I experience depression. But since being in the TM study, I am able to recover from it much faster. I'm less irritable and much easier to be around. I can handle things easier. Some people have noticed I'm a lot calmer. Others say I'm a lot less of a pushover. Maybe I'm more resilient. But the biggest effect of the study is when a stressful event occurs, I know I can take a 10- to 20-minute break from my day, close my eyes, and meditate. And in that period of time I'm usually able to level myself off.

TM has a metaphysical quality to it as well as a biological quality. There is a state of serenity that's fleeting from time to time. And it's a pretty decent feeling . . . but there's definitely a biological effect as well. There's something going on with the body here, and it's measurable. It's not just sitting and closing your eyes and then getting up out of your chair after 20 minutes. For those that say that it is a religious experience from the East, I say, "Try it for yourself before you make that kind of judgment because there is a real biological effect."

Anyone with SAD will be able to identify with the way stresses can really get you down in the winter—and how long it takes to recover from the slings and arrows of everyday life difficulties. So any technique that can help to cushion those stresses and shorten recovery time would indeed be welcome. Although there are no studies of the effects of TM (or any other form of meditation for that matter) in people with SAD, there are some compelling individual stories (a few of which I share below), as well as studies of the effects of TM on anxiety and depression in general.

TM for Anxiety and Depression

Kenneth Eppley at Stanford and his colleagues used the technique of meta-analysis to pool together 146 studies that examined trait anxiety (the tendency of people to be anxious in general). Meta-analyses are statistical techniques that researchers use to lump together a lot of different studies and come up with a single measure, called the effect size, which gives you an overall sense of the magnitude of an intervention. In behavioral sciences, an effect size is considered to be large at 0.8

unit or more, medium at 0.5 unit, and small at 0.2 unit. Eppley's meta-analysis found that TM had a large effect size in reducing state anxiety (about 0.7), compared with other stress management techniques (about 0.4).

What about depression? Although there have been no studies of TM for depression per se, depressed mood has been measured as one of the outcome variables in five controlled studies to date. In all cases the meditators showed greater improvements in depression ratings than the controls. Also, after observing some impressive—albeit anecdotal—antidepressant effects in a pilot study on the effects of TM in bipolar patients, my team and I had a brainstorming session on just how TM might alleviate depression. Here are some of the explanations that came to mind:

1. TM helps people feel calmer and improves attention. Since depressed people often experience anxiety, irritability, and poor concentration, a decrease in these symptoms might help them feel less depressed.

2. Depressed people often ruminate. TM tends to stop repetitive thoughts that loop endlessly back on themselves and may help depressed people let go of their ruminations.

3. People report TM to be a pleasant experience, look forward to their sessions, and often notice benefits soon after starting to meditate. This offers hope and a sense of having some control that is often lacking in depression. Being able to retreat twice a day to an oasis away from the continual sadness of depression allows depressed people to have a part of the day they can count on for some relief and upon which they can build a greater sense of peace.

4. Often when people are quite depressed, they are unable to refocus their thoughts in the way prescribed by CBT, a standard form of treatment for depression. TM doesn't require focusing or refocusing thoughts as it is an effortless technique that a depressed person can usually master.

5. TM may reduce the fatigue and lack of energy so common to depressed people by inducing its well-documented state of "restful alertness."

6. Depressed people often show signs of an increased stress response. For example, they experience sleep disruptions and have

elevated blood levels of glucocorticoid hormones. The well-known ability of TM to reduce stress may help correct these abnormal stress responses.

7. TM is a structured activity, and structuring the day often helps depressed people.

8. Doing something like TM, which is generally considered to have many health benefits, may improve self-esteem, which is often low in depressed people.

Could TM Help with SAD?

As I sit listening to my mantra (a very enjoyable activity), I can literally feel the stress melting away, and I continue to enjoy this benefit throughout the day. I am less likely to gun my motor for nothing, saving my energy for when I really need it. I am less likely to get riled up by the small obstacles and irritations that happen every day and more likely to say, "Let it go. It's no big deal." When I add up all these benefits, my twice-daily practice makes a huge difference to the ease with which I go about my life year round, but especially during the winter. So helpful has TM been for me that I have incorporated it into my regular anti-stress (and anti-SAD) routine and have recommended it to other SAD sufferers, many of whom have reported similar benefits.

Also consider the following stories.

Anna: A Lawyer Who Meditates

Anna is a 45-year-old leading litigation lawyer in Scotland and a single mother with a grown-up son. Although Anna makes light of her mood difficulties, saying she suffers "a wee bit from the ups and downs," she has had classical symptoms of SAD.

Anna's depressions started decades ago and are as predictable as the calendar. At the end of October, when the clocks are turned back, Anna feels "very low, very grumpy and down," and tends to "hibernate." She used to dread the winter months. She would shut herself in her apartment, wondering, "How can I get through until the light comes?"

Two years ago, a friend of hers who is a doctor in the pharmaceutical industry told her about TM. Her friend had begun to meditate and had become "a devotee." Anna knew her friend to be "a sensible girl, very scientific and cynical—not new agey at all." Yet the friend, who did not suffer from depression, "raved about it" and strongly recommended the technique to Anna, who was having trouble coping at work.

As Anna puts it, "I was so stressed out with a case at that time, you could have scraped me off the ceiling. I thought, 'What do I have to lose by doing TM, other than the money?' But I was still very skeptical." Nevertheless, here is how Anna describes the impact of TM on the course of her symptoms.

"I still don't understand the logic of it, but the technique works for me. Even though I still dislike the winter, I can cope with it. I don't have the crushing dread I used to have at the approach of winter. I used to spend a whole lot of energy getting my knickers in a twist. Now I'm not as uptight about little things, and if I start along that path, I stop myself more quickly. Even though I'm not walking on air, life has improved across the board."

Although others don't know the secret of Anna's transformation, they have certainly noticed it. According to Anna, "My opponent in a trial said, 'You're not your usual jangly self,' and my clerk asked me if I was on medication because I was doing so much better. If I miss my TM for a while, people can tell the difference even over the phone. I'm much quicker to rile, angrier, and jangly." On the other hand, when Anna does her TM regularly, she says, "Everything seems to fall into place. People are nicer to me because I am nicer to them. I get more the luck of the draw. For example, shop attendants are more likely to be helpful to me. Recently, when I traveled to a small town and was trying to find the court, I saw two parking wardens, and though they are not my favorite people—delighting as they do in issuing tickets—I asked them for directions. Not only did they show me where the court was, but they went to look for a parking space for me where I needn't pay and walked ahead of my car, showing me the way. Who has ever heard of a parking warden doing that?"

As far as the TM sessions themselves are concerned, Anna says, "I don't have wonderful experiences. I'm never in the zone." But her life is better. She realizes that "it's not about experiencing euphoria, but living a better life. It's a powerful tool in the armory of my survival, but I'm not a devotee." Anna has been "on and off antidepressants," but would prefer not to take them. She had tried a light box, "perhaps not as consistently as I should have," but didn't find that it helped her as much as TM has. She did, however, love a Caribbean trip she took one winter.

Anna is the first to acknowledge that even with TM, life is not perfect during the winters in Glasgow. "I still like watching the telly under a blanket," she says, "but I'm not staring out into the darkness, feeling doom and gloom. I still want to cuddle up and not go out into the elements, but I don't feel crushed by them."

David: SAD plus Posttraumatic Stress Disorder

One point I'd like to emphasize about people with SAD is that they often have other problems as well. Because research studies on SAD select people with as few other problems as possible, it would be easy to imagine that SAD exists in isolation. It does not. People with SAD may also suffer from anxiety disorders, bipolar disorder, and other ailments. David, currently a college student and formerly a soldier in Iraq, is such a person. I first met David when he enrolled in a research program to evaluate the potential benefits of TM for people with posttraumatic stress disorder (PTSD). He certainly qualified for that diagnosis.

He was deployed to Iraq with the 101st Airborne Division and arrived there to find "a war-torn country with blood and blown-up vehicles all over the road, the leftovers of war, along with the chemical smell of explosives that was the first thing to stick in my mind." In *Transcendence* I detail how David started developing a sense of numb detachment when he began to go out on patrol and became aware of the dangers of improvised explosive devices (IEDs) at every turn. One of these exploded, almost killing David's squad leader. Later, when David was lying in his barracks, a thousand-pound bomb went off nearby that "sounded like death" and peppered him with glass and shrapnel. According to David, "that's when I cracked."

After returning to the United States, David suffered many of the symptoms of PTSD: episodes of uncontrollable anger, disrupted sleep, exaggerated startle responses, heavy drinking, and self-destructive behavior, including single-car accidents. Flashbacks to the war zone could be triggered by ordinary stimuli. For example, smells of a gas station would remind him of the smell of burning rubber, and "all of a sudden out of nowhere, my heart started pounding. I got tense and started looking around and freaking out." His mother declared him a changed person compared to his prewar self.

TM helped David's PTSD enormously. He became calmer, settled down, and, according to his mother, became "the respectful son I knew from before." He was able to concentrate and entered college, where he is currently completing his degree in public relations.

Only after his PTSD resolved did it emerge that David had suffered from SAD since his teens. He describes his difficulties with winter as follows:

SOME PRACTICAL TIPS ABOUT TM

- The best way to find a conveniently located TM teacher is by visiting the website *www.tm.org*.

- Your local teacher should be able to tell you how to locate a free introductory lecture on TM.

- You should feel free to ask the teacher any questions pertaining to the instruction, fees, and what it is reasonable to expect from the technique.

- As with any learning process, it is important to feel comfortable with the teacher and his or her style.

- If the cost of learning is a problem, feel free to ask about scholarships or discounts for those who cannot afford the full fee. Some centers have physician- or therapist-referral programs, which offer discounted rates.

- Remember, TM can be practiced as a stand-alone technique, and there is no necessity to become involved in the TM organization in any way—unless you want to.

- An excellent Web resource on TM is *www.davidlynchfoundation.org*, which offers scholarships to people who might benefit from TM but are unable to afford it.

- For a more thorough overview of TM, I refer you to my book *Transcendence*.

I didn't like the lack of sunlight; shadows always put a damper on my moods. Winter days were a downer unless it was snowing. The full moon also seemed to help. I didn't want to be active unless the sun was out. I didn't want to get out of bed in winter, missed class, and dropped out of high school as a result of that.

This pattern continued every year until he went to Iraq, where "the winter was the best part of the year because it wasn't burning hot and it rained." Unfortunately, he was already feeling numb and suffering from PTSD, so he was not able to appreciate a sunnier winter.

The second winter after returning from Iraq David thought, "I have to get out of winter in Maryland," and went to Paraguay for 4 months. The next year, back in Maryland, he suffered again from SAD, so was back in Latin America the following winter. After returning to Maryland, he entered the TM research study and began to meditate regularly. Since then he has gone through two winters in the North with no SAD symptoms—the first time this has ever happened since his adolescence. Although he had read about SAD, he had never sought any specific treatment for it, though he is curious to try light therapy. But meditation alone seemed to take care of his symptoms. As he put it:

Although the sun wasn't shining, I felt an inner passion for what I wanted to do. The TM seems to take away the negative feelings I've experienced in winter over the years. Even though I still sometimes feel those winter feelings, they never seem to overwhelm me now. Last winter, I didn't even notice the days getting colder, nor did I succumb to the lack of sunlight.

Mindfulness

If there were fragrance
these heavy snow-flakes settling . . .
lilies on the rocks
—MATSUO BASHŌ, 17th-century haiku master

It is perhaps fitting to begin our consideration of mindfulness with this brief poem, both because of its wintry theme and because it embodies elements of mindfulness—the moment-to-moment awareness of what is going on both within oneself and outside. Bashō watches the snow-flakes settling on the rocks. They remind him of summer's lilies. He registers not only what is there but also what is not—the fragrance of the flowers.

Mindfulness is part of all Buddhist traditions. Jon Kabat-Zinn, Professor Emeritus of Medicine at the University of Massachusetts Medical School, played an important role in bringing these traditions to the West and integrating them into mainstream Western medicine. In doing so, he merged different types of Buddhist meditation into a package, which he called mindfulness. According to Rezvan Ameli, a psychologist who has taught mindfulness to personnel at the National Institutes of Health for many years, "There are two huge wings to mindfulness. One involves helping people develop moment-by-moment awareness; the other helps them develop loving-kindness." Moment-by-moment awareness is the open monitoring aspect of mindfulness mentioned earlier; loving-kindness involves focused attention. Although mindfulness has been defined by many people, a good way to think about it is "as the awareness that emerges through paying attention on purpose, in the present moment, and nonjudgmentally to things as they are" (*The Mindful Way through Depression*, p. 47).

Learning to be mindful, to observe events within one's body or the environment nonjudgmentally, on a moment-by-moment basis, can be directed to many different aspects of experience—for example, thoughts, feelings, breathing, walking, or sensory experiences. Although being mindful may sound simple, it takes practice, and expertise grows with experience and guidance. Specific exercises are geared toward helping the meditator develop these skills. One famous exercise involves learning to experience fully the taste and feel of a raisin in one's mouth. In this exercise—as in many mindfulness exercises—the experience changes from one moment to the next. Learning to observe these changes is an important aspect of the experience.

Some excellent books on the subject of mindfulness, listed in the Resources, offer exercises that can help you acquire and develop mindfulness. These books provide advice on the best posture to adopt during meditation, the best attitude to cultivate, and how to deal with problems that naturally arise (such as distraction, boredom, pain, or discomfort—physical or emotional). Many teachers recommend a gong to signal the end of a meditation session. There is a universal acceptance among those who write and teach about meditation that it cannot be learned fully just by reading. Like learning to play tennis, golf, or the piano, meditation is best learned experientially—by doing it, preferably with the help of a good teacher.

Like TM, mindfulness has been developed as a stand-alone technique and used as such in numerous research studies. Two mindfulness paradigms that have been well researched are Jon Kabat-Zinn's mindfulness-based stress reduction (MBSR) and mindfulness-based cognitive therapy (MBCT), developed by Zindel Segal, a cognitive psychologist and Professor of Psychiatry at the University of Toronto, and colleagues. MBSR combines sitting meditation, hatha yoga, and a body scan in which attention is focused sequentially on different parts of the body. I will discuss MBCT in more detail below.

How does mindfulness help depression? Many explanations have been provided, some of which I summarize below. I refer those seeking more information on this topic to *The Mindfulness Solution*, a very user-friendly book written by Ronald D. Siegel, Assistant Clinical Professor of Psychiatry at Harvard Medical School (see the Resources for more details).

1. If you tune in to your feelings moment by moment, you will realize that sadness is part of the normal spectrum of emotional colors that infuse our daily lives with variety and vibrancy. This can be difficult to appreciate for someone who associates sadness with the unremitting gloom of depression. Watching sadness come and go, or vary in quality and intensity—as mindfulness exercises teach one to do—can help someone appreciate the important distinction between sadness and depression. By normalizing sadness, mindfulness can prevent it from deepening into clinical depression.

2. Mindfulness is intentional and asks us to pay attention to present reality, which then allows us to make choices instead of being unaware, or being lost in thought, or on "automatic pilot." For a depressed person, just recognizing you have choices can be helpful. In fact, these elements of mindfulness—being aware or becoming aware—of what is going on in the mind and the body are emphasized in many forms of therapy.

3. By trying to avoid pain we can make painful feelings worse. This is in fact one of the Buddha's cardinal insights—his "First Noble

Truth." Mindfulness can help us face that pain and see it for what it is. Traditional therapies also recognize that tendencies to push away unwelcome thoughts and feelings (so-called "defense mechanisms") may actually make one's problems worse.

4. Sometimes we judge our feelings harshly, thereby making the pain worse. Mindfulness teaches us to look at our emotions as they are, without judging them. Seeing these emotions for what they are can be a relief—and lessen their impact on our overall mood.

5. We can also tend to judge our choices—or planned choices—harshly, seeing them as foolish, misguided, or inadequate. Whether these choices are good or bad, in judging them you are often comparing yourself to some standard—asking "Why can't I be the person I'm supposed to be?"—which often creates a sense of shame or blame. The loving-kindness or self-compassion facet of mindfulness meditation can help you suffer less from the barbs of your inner critic.

6. Finding missing emotions can be helpful—for example, you may be sad *and* angry. Tuning in to your different feelings can give you a greater sense of variety in your emotional life—as opposed to monolithic depression.

7. Mindfulness can help you identify negative cognitions, as described in Chapter 9. By setting time aside and practicing exercises that help develop your ability to focus on your feelings, sensations *and* thoughts, you are more likely to identify these negative cognitions—a critical first step in all cognitive-behavioral interventions.

8. In contrast to rumination, mindfulness is present-centered and doesn't take us down paths of an imagined future or a disquieting past. Mindfulness interrupts the cycle of rumination that often accompanies the downward cycle of your mood.

Treating SAD with Mindfulness

Mindfulness-based techniques have been found to alleviate depression and anxiety. One recent meta-analysis that considered 39 studies involving 1,140 participants found moderate effect sizes for improving anxiety (0.63) and depression (0.59) for the group as a whole, but large effect sizes when they considered people with diagnosed anxiety and mood disorders (approximately 0.95 for both groups).

These techniques have never been tested for SAD per se, nor had any of the experts I consulted specifically treated any people with SAD with mindfulness. Luckily, however, with the help of the SAD Association of Great Britain (SADA), I was able to locate a few people with SAD who have benefited greatly by treating their winter symptoms with different types of mindfulness exercises. Here are their stories.

Helen: Mindful across the Seasons

Helen is a retired biology lecturer in her late 60s who lives in the north of England. She suffered from severe SAD until the late 1990s, when she heard a radio program on SAD and decided to do something about it. Before then she had felt very low during the winter months and had trouble concentrating and dealing with friends and family. She recalls days when she felt so down that she would lie on the floor sobbing, though she never allowed herself to miss work on account of her depression.

After hearing about SAD on the radio, Helen began to use a light box, which made a significant difference in her ability to function. She has also tried the herbal antidepressant St. John's wort, which has helped during the worst part of winter. Interestingly, although some people have complained of sore eyes when using the combination of light therapy and St. John's wort (which is a known photosensitizer), this combination has not caused Helen any problems.

Toward the end of the 1990s, Helen also became interested in Buddhism and began to practice two forms of Buddhist meditation each day—first she uses breathing meditation to calm herself down, then Vipassana (insight) meditation. Once a week, she adds loving-kindness meditation to her regular practice. (As noted at the beginning of the chapter, Vipassana meditation is a form of open monitoring and loving-kindness is a form of focused attention, both of which are part of mindfulness.) Her meditation has taught Helen to "observe the rising and passing of states of mind." She adds, "The Buddhist approach that it passes—that all things pass—helps you reach a state of equanimity." Others have commented that she seems more tranquil since starting to meditate.

Helen sees light therapy and meditation as complementary. In the winter, she generally sits by the light box first while eating breakfast, then does her meditation. She has found it too difficult to concentrate on meditation before doing light therapy. In general, I advise people to do the same. As we know, light therapy is often most effective if done first thing in the morning and, as with Helen, doing it may actually improve your meditation.

Helen still doesn't feel as good in winter as she does in summer, but she feels *much* better than she felt before starting light therapy and meditation.

Marjorie: Mindful Walks in Kew Gardens

According to the *Time Out* guide to London, "Kew's lush, landscaped beauty represents the pinnacle of our national gardening obsession." Like many other tourists, I have wandered along the paths and sampled the visual delights of these famous botanical gardens. Marjorie, an art teacher in her early 60s, is fortunate enough to live around the corner from these gardens. Besides her art teaching, Marjorie has home-schooled her developmentally disabled son, now 19 years old, who is easily overloaded with sensory stimuli and needs one-on-one tutoring.

Marjorie has had SAD for as long as she can remember, though she only recognized she had this disorder when she was about 40. She has always been very depressed in winter and has always broken up with partners in February. She has tried using a light box, but it causes her to have "a migraine aura—funny eye symptoms that involve seeing jagged semi-circles" to one side of her visual field. She has benefited a lot, however, from using a dawn simulator and increasing the indoor lighting in her home. She has never tried antidepressants because she is very sensitive to drugs in general, including caffeine and alcohol.

Marjorie has always been attracted to meditation. As a student, she learned TM, which she found "very powerful." Like many others, however, she allowed her practice to lapse. She has always found sitting meditation difficult because she is constantly disrupted when at home. Her solution has been to embrace the walking meditation popularized by Thich Nhat Hanh, a Vietnamese Buddhist monk and author. And where better for Marjorie to practice this than in Kew Gardens?

As she walks, assuming "the half-smile of the Buddha," Marjorie counts her steps and her breathing. She also says things like "I've arrived, I'm home, in the here, in the now, I'm solid, I'm free, in the ultimate I dwell." Sometimes she sits down on one of the park benches and counts as she breathes. These exercises help Marjorie relax and get rid of her obsessive thoughts.

I asked Marjorie whether it may not simply be walking outdoors in beautiful surroundings that has such a salutary effect on her mood. She discounts that explanation:

> *It really feels better than simply walking. I used to walk around Kew Gardens but would come back feeling more negative—as though I had been rehearsing and amplifying my negative thinking during the walk. I would come back feeling more wound up both emotionally and physically—until I began the walking meditation.*

Marjorie also incorporates mindfulness into her daily life, for example, when washing the dishes.

> *I note the color of things, my feelings, the movements of my body. It grounds and calms me. It gets me out of my head.*

Like many others, Marjorie uses several different techniques to get her through the winter—but mindfulness meditation has been an important part of her anti-SAD regimen.

Loving-Kindness Compassion

Loving-kindness compassion, a form of meditation that Helen practices once a week after meditating to her breath, is often considered one aspect of mindfulness, as mentioned earlier. Boston psychologist Christopher Germer, author of *The Mindful Path to Self-Compassion* (see the Resources), both practices loving-kindness compassion personally and recommends the technique to his patients. The essence of this form of meditation is to use mindfulness exercises to tune in to your inner thoughts and feelings, then to give yourself messages of loving-kindness and compassion. In distinguishing between these two emotions, Germer quotes the Dalai Lama:

> *Loving-kindness is the wish for all beings to be happy, and compassion is the wish for all beings to be free from suffering. And that distinction*

shakes out differently in meditation. For example, if you're practicing compassion meditation, you actually meditate in response to naturally arising suffering, or you just drop into your body and discover all this stress and strain that we carry in our bodies all the time. And then, when we make an actual visceral contact with—or develop an awareness of— that stress and strain, we give ourselves loving-kindness in the form of: "May I be safe?" "May I be peaceful?" "May I be kind to myself?"

Why is it so important, I asked Germer, to phrase things in just that way? Here's how he responded:

The reason is that we're actually cultivating goodwill and we're not directly cultivating good feelings, because we're not trying to manipulate our moment-to-moment experience. In other words, if we're feeling unpeaceful, and we issue positive affirmations to ourselves—"I'm peaceful," "I'm peaceful," "I'm peaceful"—that can make us feel even worse (because deep down we're not feeling peaceful). So what we try to do instead is to incline the heart, or cultivate an attitude toward ourselves while we're suffering—just like a mother with a child who has the flu. The mother doesn't say, "Knock it off, kid. You can't have the flu; get up and go to school." Nor does the mother blame herself because the child has the flu. The mother will sit with the child, and maybe put a cool towel on the child's forehead. Basically the way we attend to somebody who's sick until the sickness passes is the same way we attend to ourselves when we're suffering until the suffering passes. We're not trying to drive it away. That's why we say, "May I." It's an inclination of heart; it's cultivating goodwill rather than good feeling.

Germer believes that his approach to therapy—mindful self-compassion—is especially helpful for depressed people, who experience significant degrees of shame. Germer describes a young man who consulted him because of panic attacks, about which he had marked feelings of shame. Germer encouraged the man to meditate on thoughts of self-compassion, such as "May I be safe," "May I be peaceful," "May I accept myself as I am," "May I accept the conditions of my life as I am." Eventually, the young man reached the point where he realized, "This is not my fault. I didn't ask to have panic attacks. It's not my fault that

I have them." According to Germer, this was a profound transformational experience for him.

It is not difficult to see how some of Germer's insights could be applied to people with SAD. I often hear from my patients with SAD about their feelings of shame or embarrassment when they have difficulty coping in the winter and are unable to keep up with their work or domestic and personal responsibilities. Many have also been too embarrassed to bring a light box in to work because of what others might think. Perhaps Germer's approach would help them feel less ashamed about something that is, after all, not their fault. For more information about Germer, I refer you to his website (see the Resources), which has free downloadable meditation exercises for you to sample.

Mindfulness-Based Cognitive Therapy

Mindfulness in the form of MBCT has been highly successful in preventing relapses in people with recurrent depressions. The program was developed by Zindel Segal, a cognitive psychologist and Professor of Psychiatry at the University of Toronto, and colleagues. MBCT combines cognitive-behavioral techniques with sitting meditation, hatha yoga, and a body scan in which attention is focused sequentially on different parts of the body. According to Segal, MBCT helps patients develop "meta-awareness skills," which enhance "the ability to observe their experiences, to watch thoughts as mental events and not to be completely identified with them."

Segal explains further:

> These meta-awareness skills have been described in psychotherapy as adopting an observing stance on experience, an observing ego. So that if you're having critical thoughts, you might say to yourself, "Oh, critical thoughts are here. I'm thinking very critically of myself right now," rather than being completely consumed by what the thoughts are saying about you. And this, I think, gives people the ability to work with that material very differently.

Segal emphasizes that at this time, as far as treatment of depression is concerned, MBCT should be recommended only to help prevent relapse because there is evidence that regular CBT is far stronger as a treatment for acute depression. He points out that "in speaking to people who have practiced mindfulness for many years and have a history of depression, they find it very difficult to muster the concentration and attention capacities required for this practice in the middle of a depression where those very faculties are compromised." For preventing depression relapses, however, MBCT appears to be highly effective, yielding results that were comparable to antidepressant medications in one recent study.

Since SAD is by definition a recurrent and predictable form of depression, MBCT would certainly be worth trying for people with SAD—especially since the cognitive-behavioral elements that are part of the program have themselves been found to help people with SAD *and* protect against subsequent episodes. Those with a history of SAD could learn about MBCT in the spring and summer and have their program in place by the time winter arrives. For those interested in finding out more about this technique, I recommend the highly readable book *The Mindful Way through Depression* by Zindel and colleagues, which is listed in the Resources.

Closing Thoughts

In revising *Winter Blues* for its fourth edition, this chapter on meditation for SAD is the only entirely new chapter I have added. Although as yet there are no controlled studies of any form of meditation for SAD, I hope that after reading this chapter you will share my excitement about the potential of the forms of meditation discussed here as valuable treatment options. Throughout the natural world, winter is a time for slowing down and withdrawal from the frenetic activities of the rest of the year. Perhaps we can learn something from other species and incorporate deep physical and emotional rest into our winter routine. If you choose to do so, you can use the ideas and observations in this chapter (along with the resources listed at the back of the book) to help you add meditation to your winter program, just as Anna, David, Helen, Marjorie, and I have done.

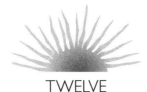

TWELVE

A Step-by-Step Guide through the Revolving Year

▶ What does the annual cycle of your seasonality look like?

▶ How can you plan ahead for your toughest months?

▶ What can you do to take advantage of your easiest months?

▶ How do you handle the winter holidays?

With some variation from year to year, the seasons revolve in a certain predictable rhythm. This is a fact that is impossible to ignore, especially for those whose mood seems so closely tied to that rhythm. But with the worst of your SAD symptoms occurring in the darkest months, it's easy to forget that you have specific responses to the other times of year as well. Being able to predict and plan for those responses can help you travel through the revolving year more smoothly and productively. In this chapter, I examine these predictable changes and encourage you to do the same, examining your year as a whole and planning accordingly. Forewarned is forearmed, as they say, and nowhere is this more true than in understanding the predictable cycle of your seasonal changes.

*W*hen we think of the changing seasons, many different images
come to mind. One image that has stayed with me since my colleagues and I published the first description of the syndrome of SAD is
that of a staircase. We asked the first 19 patients with SAD studied at
the NIMH to think back over the course of their seasonal problems and
note the months when they typically experienced their winter symptoms. Figure 9, reproduced from the initial publication that resulted
from that study, illustrates when that first group of patients experienced their symptoms in relation to the day length in Rockville, Maryland, which is at the latitude where the study occurred.

As you can see, some difficulties began in September, and the fre-

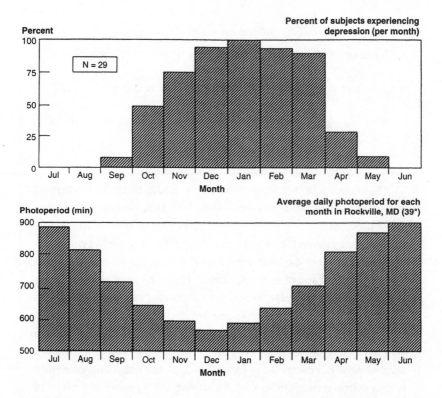

**FIGURE 9. Relationship between symptoms of SAD and length of day (pho-
toperiod).** From Rosenthal et al. (1984). This figure is in the public domain.

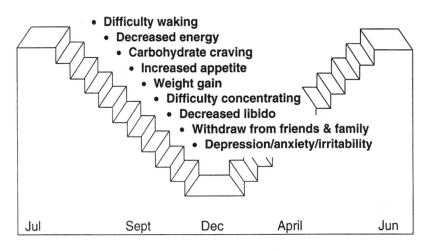

FIGURE 10. Symptoms of SAD.

quency of symptoms rose progressively over the next 4 months, reaching a peak in January, remaining high in February and March, and then declining sharply in April and May. There is a correspondence between the frequency of symptoms and day length, with symptoms increasing as day length decreases toward the winter solstice and the reverse occurring as the days lengthen once again. I have often thought of the lower part of the graph as a staircase leading downward as mood declines with the waning light and then leading upward again as mood improves with the return of the sun. If you look at the graph carefully, you will note that there is not an exact correspondence between day length and symptom frequency. Symptoms remain at high levels through January and February even though the days are getting longer through those months. We believe this happens because January and February are very dark and cloudy months, at least in Maryland, and even though the days are getting longer, the actual amount of sunlight perceived is often at its lowest after the winter solstice.

It is helpful to consider the typical progression of the symptoms of SAD using this image of a staircase. Although people differ as to when they get their symptoms over the course of the year—and indeed what symptoms they get—a very typical progression is shown in Figure 10.

As you can see, problems with mood do not usually occur early in the progression. Instead, the earliest problems usually involve sleep and energy difficulties, followed by appetite and weight changes, problems with concentrating, and reduced sex drive and socializing. It is often only after these changes are under way that people begin to feel depressed, anxious, and irritable.

Whenever I see someone with SAD, one of the first things I do is establish the pattern of the person's annual cycle:

- When do the first symptoms occur?
- What are these symptoms, and how do they progress through the revolving seasons?
- When does the person begin to emerge from the depression, and what are the other seasons like?

One such person is Keith, a social scientist in his late 30s with a history of SAD going back at least 22 years. Considering that he studied economics and law at the finest Ivy League universities, it is curious that he went so long without recognizing the nature of his problem and seeking help for it. He attributes this delay to two factors. First, he had a friend, a woman with debilitating SAD, who would routinely gain 10 to 12 pounds each winter, sleep 10 to 12 hours a day, and suffer terribly until spring arrived.

> *Establishing the pattern of your annual cycle helps you plan for the coming year to make it less troublesome and more enjoyable than the previous one.*

He contrasted the relative mildness of his own symptoms with hers and failed to recognize that they had the same condition, but to different degrees. Second, he had been strongly influenced by psychological and sociological schools of thought, which seek to explain behavior as a result of human interactions rather than as a biological effect of the physical world.

Once Keith was able to make the paradigm shift from a psychological to a biological model, he was able to apply his intellect to understanding his problem and communicate this to me in a way that was so illuminating and compelling that I have chosen his story to illustrate the predictable effects of the changing seasons on our minds and our bodies.

The History of Your Annual Cycle

In one of his first visits to me, Keith produced the graph in Figure 11. The graph shows the typical pattern of his annual mood changes. He thought back over the previous 10 years and assigned numbers to each month, with higher numbers corresponding to when he was in good spirits, lower numbers to when he was in his depressed periods, and the midline corresponding to when he was in an even mood. In producing this graph, he created a valuable template for us to use in planning his forthcoming year's treatment. In fact, I first saw Keith in the spring, and based on the graph, we both decided that it would not be necessary for us to meet until the following September after Labor Day, when we would plan his course of action for the following winter.

If you suffer from SAD, I encourage you to map out the history of your own annual cycle. Figure 12 provides a grid that asks you to rate your mood for each month over the last 5 years. If you can't remember that far back, 3 years will probably do just fine. If you have moved to a different latitude or climatic region in the last few years, the exercise

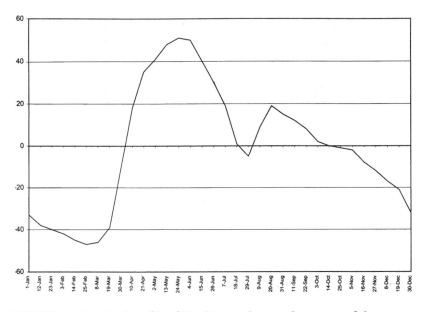

FIGURE 11. A typical profile of Keith's moods over the course of the year.

Scale: +50 = The best I've ever felt
             0 = Even mood
           −50 = The worst I've ever felt

Year	July	Aug.	Sept.	Oct.	Nov.	Dec.	Jan.	Feb.	Mar.	April	May	June
Last year												
2 years ago												
3 years ago												
4 years ago												
5 years ago												
Average												

FIGURE 12. Monthly mood ratings to help you develop numbers to graph your seasonal profile. *From Winter Blues* (4th ed.). Copyright 2013 by Norman E. Rosenthal.

may be less reliable since your seasonal pattern of mood and behavior will tend to change with latitude and climate. Once you have put numbers in all the squares of the grid, you should average the numbers for each month and enter them in the graph provided in Figure 13. That will give you a picture of your own annual cycle, which will help you plan out the coming year. (If you don't want to mark up your book, feel free to photocopy the forms or download them from the book's page at *www.guilford.com*)

I recommend that you purchase a special journal or calendar for the year and mark in it some of the key points in your own annual cycle: when your mood begins to slide, when it crosses the midline, when it reaches its low point, when it begins to recover, and so on. As we look further into the predictable changes that the year brings, there will be other days and dates that you might want to mark on this calendar and that may help you with your planning. Be sure that there is room in the journal for you to make notes as well.

THE GENERAL PRINCIPLES OF SAD TREATMENT

- Plan in advance.

- Start treating early.

- Begin with the simplest treatment.

- Layer treatments one on top of the other.

- Peel off the layers of treatment one by one as the days begin to lengthen again.

Once you understand your own seasonal pattern, you can consider how to incorporate the treatments described in earlier chapters into an overall treatment plan. The image of a staircase can help you consider how treatments can be sequenced. Figure 14 shows how I might sequence the treatments for someone with severe SAD, though most people do not require all the treatments shown and differ as to when they may need different treatments. In general, I try to get away with as little treatment as possible to achieve my goal, which is the

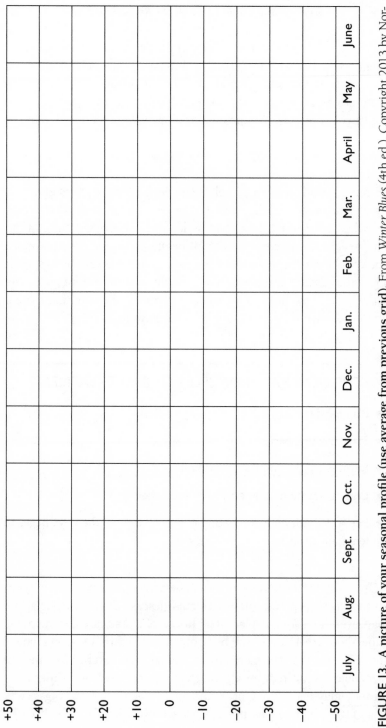

FIGURE 13. A picture of your seasonal profile (use average from previous grid). From *Winter Blues* (4th ed.). Copyright 2013 by Norman E. Rosenthal.

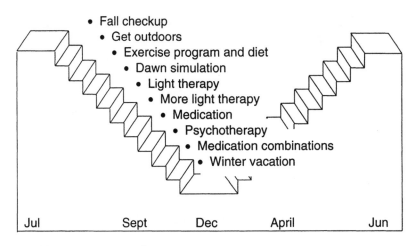

- Fall checkup
  - Get outdoors
    - Exercise program and diet
      - Dawn simulation
        - Light therapy
          - More light therapy
            - Medication
              - Psychotherapy
                - Medication combinations
                  - Winter vacation

| Jul | Sept | Dec | April | Jun |

FIGURE 14. Treatment of SAD.

maintenance of good mood, energy level, and functioning throughout the winter months.

Treating Keith

In treating Keith, I followed the diagram to some degree. I suggested that he be sure to get as much outdoor light as possible and start to use a dawn simulator in September. In mid-October, which is where he usually crosses his midline and moves into the depressed region, I suggested he begin light therapy for about 15 minutes in the morning and 15 minutes in the evening. It had an immediate effect of buoying him up, making him feel safe and warm. It also made him "very jumpy." Within a few minutes of starting therapy, his pulse went up to 90 beats per minute, his nasal passages dried up, and he developed headaches, but after 2 weeks these side effects stabilized and he fell into a more comfortable pattern of using the light. It is quite unusual to experience such marked side effects so quickly after starting light therapy.

This is how Keith describes the first winter of using lights.

On the one hand, mentally and emotionally I deployed all my emotional reserve to prepare for the onslaught of winter—all the signs were there—my memories of these winters were so profound that I spent a good deal of the fall on guard. On the whole, I had the sense that I still dipped and declined, still slipped behind and coasted for a while—though it was not a depression but a recession, as an economist would say. But all the while I felt that there was a lifeline, that I was wearing a harness, a climber's rope—that if I fell, there would be a stop to the fall that would catch me long before I hit bottom—that there was a safety net.

Many of the symptoms returned in kind but to a lesser degree. Tastes definitely changed—both musical and food tastes—but I never became monotonic. I don't believe I ever had trouble getting out of bed during the winter. I used a dawn simulator; more important, I think, I opened the shutters at night for the first time in 20 years. But the dawn simulator has been a balm. Many times I would wake up before the alarm, which would have been inconceivable in years past.

This winter I had to be in charge of the most high-profile and stress-ful piece of work in my life, the preparation of which coincided with what have been the traditionally worst weeks of my life—from the first weeks of November to the middle of February—and I never faltered. Without treatment I would still have managed but would have had no energy for anything else; that was not the case this year. I managed to get to the movies, go to parties, and even host a dinner party.

There were a couple of bad spells, but I could almost always link those to not having done the lights for several days or critically depleting my energy through inadequate sleep or excessive stress.

The one thing that was very much absent this year was the feeling of being trapped in a tunnel and the sense that time has significantly pro-longed itself. It felt as though May was a world away in the past; this year that long stretching out of time—to the point of feeling that every day did not get you closer to the spring—did not happen. The year kept its shape.

I remember waking up on a Saturday in early January, looking at the calendar, seeing that February ended on a Saturday, and thinking to myself, "Eight weeks; all right, here we go," and being surprised at how fast the time went.

Predictable Markers of the Revolving Year and What You Can Do about Them

Although the year has a certain rhythm to it, the exact nature of that rhythm will differ from person to person and, to some extent, from year to year. Take some time to think about your year as a whole and note the important markers: points when you can expect seasonal effects as well as the timing of predictable events such as a vacation; the dates when the children get out of school, go off to summer camp, or come home from college; deadlines; and major life events or stresses. You might want to record these in your journal or calendar so that you can be sure to take them into account when you plan your year.

Summertime

To paraphrase the famous lyrics from *Porgy and Bess*, during summertime, the living is easy for most people with SAD. To be sure, some people have predictable summer difficulties, and this may not be as exhilarating a time as spring or fall. If you look over Keith's annual profile, you will see a small downward notch in midsummer. Writers and artists say that summer is a less creative time for them than spring or autumn, according to Kay Redfield Jamison, who has studied creativity and its relationship to mood disorders. Some people suffer from summer depressions, others from summer hypomania, and yet others do not emerge completely from their winter depression even after summer arrives. But for most of us, summer is a carefree time, when we want to get away, to play and forget that winter was ever here and will ever come back again. But for those of us who, like the fabled grasshopper, would prefer to play all summer long, here are some pointers that could come in handy when the dark days of winter arrive.

- Don't spend all your vacation time during the summer. Save at least some of it for the winter, when you will need it more.

- If you have a major task to undertake, such as changing your job, moving, or relocating to another city, do so in the summer, when you have more energy.

- If you do move in summer, check to make sure that your new house, apartment, or office is well illuminated all year round. It might be bright during the summer but dark as a dungeon during the winter.

- This might be a good time to plan for the winter, though in reality most people wait until the end of summer to do so.

September—The Beginning of Fall

Labor Day is often a reliable marker of the beginning of fall, in both the culture and the natural world, even though the formal beginning of the season is the autumnal equinox some 2 to 3 weeks later. In September, some people are beginning to feel the onset of their winter symptoms—changes in appetite, sleep patterns, or energy level—while others are still fine at this time.

No matter how mild or severe your winter difficulties usually are, I recommend that you undertake a fall checkup. Consider taking the following steps:

- Purchase necessary lighting equipment. If the light tubes in a light box are more than two years old, consider replacing them.
- Put your exercise and dietary program in place.
- Do what you can to keep predictable stresses to a manageable level over the winter.
- Plan one or more winter breaks in a southern locale—if feasible and affordable.
- Inform family members, friends, and, when appropriate, colleagues or associates that you are soon going to enter your less sociable season and become less dynamic than you have been during the summer. Engage their support ahead of time where appropriate. Obviously, judgment needs to be exercised in deciding when it would be helpful for others at work to be informed about your seasonal difficulties and when you are better off keeping this to yourself.
- Consider consulting appropriate professionals—such as a therapist, physician, or dietitian—so that they are on board at the beginning of the winter.
- Get outdoors and enjoy the beauty that nature has to offer at this time of year.
- Be sure to keep your bedroom shades up and your shutters open so that you can benefit from the first rays of morning sunlight.
- Start using your dawn simulator to offset the effects of the shortening days. The autumnal equinox is that time of year when days are shortening most rapidly.
- Look ahead to the section on December that follows and also

see the suggestions about stress management on pages 186–188. Make a list of things that need to be done for the holidays and do as much as possible ahead of time. This can include purchasing, writing, and addressing cards; assembling decorations for the Christmas tree or buying Hanukkah candles; buying gifts early; or informing people that this holiday season is going to be a bit different from others (that is, it will involve less work for you).

October, November, and the Daylight Savings Time Change

In the North, October is a variable month. There are still some fine days, but winter is beginning to assert itself. Like Keith, many people with SAD need to start using their light box during this month. I usually recommend that people start with short durations of light exposure—for example, 15 minutes once or twice a day. As the month progresses, this duration may need to be increased, but it is always wise to use your own internal state as a guide to how much light you need.

The first Sunday in November is when the clocks are usually set back an hour, a transition that often causes difficulties for people with SAD. For them, the extra hour of darkness in the evening is a heavy price to pay for the extra hour of light in the morning, which they are often unable to benefit from fully since they are generally asleep or indoors at that hour. At this time it may be useful to:

- Initiate a program of morning walks to take advantage of the extra morning sunlight.
- Increase the amount of evening light therapy to deal with the extra hour of darkness at that time while continuing to use light therapy in the morning.
- Consider writing your holiday cards and doing some of your holiday shopping and planning before you feel overwhelmed by the effects of the short, dark days.
- Consider doing bulk shopping for nonperishable goods to save yourself the effort later on.

In the northern United States and northern Europe, November seems to be the month when people with SAD really begin to feel bad.

Their general sentiments toward this month were well expressed by two great American writers: Herman Melville in *Moby-Dick* and Henry Adams, the famous chronicler of American life. Here are their thoughts about November:

> Whenever I find myself growing grim about the mouth; whenever it is a damp, drizzly November in my soul; whenever I find myself involuntarily pausing before coffin warehouses, and bringing up the rear of every funeral I meet; and especially whenever my hypos get such an upper hand of me, that it requires a strong moral principle to prevent me from knocking people's hats off—then, I account it high time to get to sea as soon as I can. (Herman Melville, *Moby-Dick*)

> Dear Boy:
>
> I sit down to begin you a letter, not because I have received one since my last, but because it is one of the dankest, foggiest, and dismalest of November nights, and, as usual when the sun does not shine, I am as out of sorts as a man may haply be, and yet live through it. . . . This season of the year grinds the very soul out of me. My nerves lose their tone, my teeth ache, and my courage falls to the bottomless bottom of infinitude. Death stalks about me, and the whole of Gray's grisly train, and I am afraid of them, not because life is an object, but because my nerves are upset. I would give up all my pleasures willingly if I could only be a mouse, and sleep three months at a time. Well! one can't have life as one would, but if I ever take too much laudanum, the coroner's jury may bring in a verdict of willful murder against the month of November. (Henry Adams, letter to Charles Milnes Gaskell, November 1869)

Some years ago a coroner in England did in fact bring in a verdict of murder against the month of November, or rather, the cause of death was given as SAD. The victim was an Englishwoman who had just returned to England in November from a vacation in some sunny place when she became overwhelmed by symptoms of severe SAD, which drove her to suicide. It is always hard to think about someone taking his or her own life, but this is especially so when the condition in question is completely treatable. No one should have to feel so cornered by SAD that suicide appears to be the only way out.

The following guidelines may help steer you through this difficult month.

- By now, most people need light therapy regularly. While the daily duration of therapy needed is variable, it is not at all unusual for people to need 30 to 45 minutes in the morning and the evening.
- Be sure to maintain your exercise program. If you let it slip now, it may be hard to retrieve it through the rest of the winter. Light therapy will help you stick to your exercise routine. Try to keep up with your morning walks on bright fall days.
- You may need medications at this time, but check with your doctor before starting them. I do not recommend, for example, that you simply pick up last year's medicine bottle and start taking the leftovers, calling your doctor only when you have run out of medications.
- Watch out for holiday foods and eating patterns. Once the weight creeps on this early in the season, it can careen out of control in the months to come. See Chapter 8 for more information about this.

December and the Holiday Season

People with SAD often regard December and the holiday season with mixed feelings. It is no coincidence, of course, that major holidays, such as Christmas and Hanukkah, occur around the winter solstice and involve the kindling of light—the Yule log, the Hanukkah menorah, the Christmas tree. Rituals of renewal at the approach of the New Year, prayers for the return of the sun, and the need for holiday cheer, which is enhanced by illumination, feasting, and drinking, come together in the modern celebration of the winter festivals as they have for centuries. Even as people with SAD may struggle to keep up with the chores and expectations that attend the holidays, so their spirits may be buoyed up by the great carnival that overtakes our society at this time of year.

From the vantage point of the declining light, all the same principles that operated in November continue and all the same advice applies. Fortunately, less is often expected of people at work during the holidays, which can be a great relief to someone suffering from SAD. On the other hand, it can be a difficult season for those in charge at home, who not only have many additional chores and duties associated with the holidays but also feel an extra sense of responsibility for creating a convivial and joyous atmosphere. When you are feeling fatigued, withdrawn, and sad, that is a particularly tall order.

Advice to Celebration Planners Who Struggle with the Winter Holidays

If you're the person in your household who usually takes on the primary responsibility for planning holiday celebrations and handling many of the preparations, it's important to give yourself a break at this tough time of year:

- Now is the time to benefit from some of the plans put in place earlier in the season (see September, p. 264).
- Explain to your family why this season is difficult for someone with SAD; that you will be able to do only a limited number of things toward making the holidays special. Enlist their help and support. Remind yourself and them that what is really special about the holidays is being together and enjoying one another's company. Sometimes this is easiest to do and works best if the holiday season is kept relatively simple.
- Consider not making the winter festival the one when you do most of the work; for example, you might make less fuss over Christmas or Hanukkah and put on an extra-good Easter egg hunt or have Passover at your place next spring.
- Get as much help as possible. For example, maybe there is a service that delivers a Christmas tree to you. Paying someone to help clean the house at this time may be the best holiday gift you can give yourself. Divide up the work and organize the family to do different chores.
- Consider going to a restaurant for at least one of the holiday meals.
- Actively work on not feeling guilty; remember, you never asked to get SAD.
- Consider increasing the amount of light therapy or other treatments you are receiving to help you get through the holiday season.

Travel over the Holidays

If you need to leave home for more than a day or two from December through February, it is usually very important to take your light therapy apparatus (dawn simulator, light box, or light visor) with you. You will probably bridle at the inconvenience, but believe me, in most cases it is well worth it.

Despite his reservations, one young man with SAD decided to take his light box with him to his fiancée's home over the Christmas break. He found his fiancée's family to be interested in and accepting of his predicament, and more important, he was able to enjoy his time with her and with them.

One problem with successful treatment of SAD is that you can easily forget you have the condition at all. I have made this error myself, most egregiously on a trip to Tromsö, a city north of the Arctic Circle, where I was invited to chair a conference on SAD during the depths of winter. I thought that I could manage without the lights for the 3 or 4 days of the conference and arrived in the city during its legendary dark days, when the sun does not rise above the horizon. The very day I landed there, I felt the energy drain out of my system, like blood running out of my veins, and all I wanted to do was to lie on my bed and stare at the ceiling.

The conference organizers informed me that it would be a day or more before they could have a light box sent in, but I was fortunate to be bailed out by Jennifer Eastwood, head of SADA, a presenter at the conference who had made all the necessary arrangements to have a light box installed in her room from day one. This she was gracious enough to share with me. As I sat in front of the box, I felt energy returning to me within the hour and all of a sudden was buzzing with excitement at being in this famous northern city at a conference devoted exclusively to SAD and its treatments.

The moral of the story is: If I can forget my light box in a place and at a time when I desperately needed it, so can you. Don't deny the extent of your SAD symptoms and forget the degree to which you are being buoyed up by your light therapy, and be sure to see that you have adequate light exposure when you travel.

The Holiday Blues and SAD

For therapists in clinical practice it is not unusual to see some feelings of sadness around the time of the holidays. Although this is a time when people are supposed to be happy, and many are, for some the expected happiness does not arrive. Lonely people, people without family or friends, and people who grew up in dysfunctional families and have unpleasant associations with the holidays simply can't achieve the ideal that many commercial images of the holidays portray. Obviously, having SAD can only increase the unhappiness of people who also feel the holiday blues.

How can you tell which problem is plaguing you? The holiday blues are really quite distinct from SAD in that people with SAD are suffering from a clinical depression that arises largely from their special biology, whereas the holiday blues involve sadness that arises out of psychological conflicts. SAD typically lasts for several months, whereas the holiday blues are usually confined to the holiday season. Finally, people with SAD typically experience a variety of physical changes—for example, in eating, sleeping, energy level, and daily functioning. Most people who are simply reacting to Christmas or the holidays do not generally show these changes.

Although a number of studies have tried to document the holiday blues by examining, for example, the frequency of visits to the emergency room for psychiatric help, or admissions to psychiatric units during the holiday season, it has been an elusive entity to nail down. In fact, one study showed that presentations to psychiatric emergency rooms decreased in the few days before major holidays and increased in the few days afterward. It is as though people did not want to spoil their holidays by going to the emergency room, so they waited until the holidays were over before doing so.

Despite the absence of studies demonstrating the existence of the holiday blues, they certainly do exist. I have never been more aware of this than during one holiday season when I was asked to participate in a radio program about the holiday blues along with a few other professionals. The radio station typically played music that appealed to a teenage audience, which might have accounted for why those who called in were predominantly young. Many of them had heartbreaking stories, of being alone over the holidays, of not having the kind of holidays they imagined other families had, of broken relationships and other sources of grief, experienced with the intensity that is perhaps unique to adolescence. Hearing these stories one after the other was quite moving. I was impressed in particular by one young caller who described the great pain and hardship in her life around the holidays. During a commercial break, one of my colleagues on the show acknowledged that the distressed young lady was in fact her daughter. She said sadly that she had tried to do whatever she could to help her through the holidays, apparently to no avail. The incident helped me realize how complex and difficult the holiday blues can be—sometimes for the whole family.

There is no reason, of course, why people might not suffer from both SAD and the holiday blues. The many chores and activities that surround the holidays pose an extra burden to those with SAD. In addition, since SAD often runs in families, the holiday season may trigger memories of a parent who was unable to cope at that time of year and might have tried to do so by withdrawing, being irritable, or getting drunk.

If the holidays are a recurrent source of pain and difficulty for you, seek out a therapist to help you anticipate and deal with them.

Only when you've come to understand your difficulties with the holidays and have found a way to cope with them can they become a time of genuine celebration. Look beyond the commercial elements of the holidays—as well as the duties, chores, and conventional activities that attend the season—and try to seize what is great about it—kindness, community, relaxation, and generosity of spirit. Since charity begins at home, start by being kind to yourself and don't overload yourself with social and other holiday responsibilities. That will help you be more available to yourself and others at this time of year.

Anniversary Reactions

One factor that can affect the way you feel at any time of year is the anniversary of some sad event that occurred at that time in your past. When such an anniversary comes during a season that is already difficult, it can compound the hardship of the season.

In contrast to the symptoms of SAD, these anniversary reactions usually occur specifically around the date of the anniversary and do not typically last for weeks or months. They do make life more difficult, though. One of my patients, a professional, would recall the anniversary of her mother's suicide in October many years before. She anticipated her memories of the shocking details for weeks in advance and it quite shook her for much of October. It was very important for her to acknowledge and understand the power that this memory continued to have over her as a source of pain distinct from her SAD. On the other hand, I have seen people with SAD try to explain their recurrent winter symptoms purely as a reaction to the anniversary of some sad event in the past, which is an unsatisfactory approach both in terms of accounting for the full extent of the SAD symptoms and in planning a proper treatment plan for them.

- If you know that a certain time of year brings up painful memories, make a note of this date in your journal and planner.
- Let friends, family, and other supportive people know that the date is approaching and seek extra support from them at this time. They probably won't know how difficult the memories are for you unless you tell them.
- Plan activities that help you come to terms with the pain of the memory. For example, you may want to visit a special place that reminds you of a lost loved one in the company of a supportive and loving person.
- Recognize that you might not function as well over the days around the anniversary and cut yourself some slack.
- You will deal best with the anniversary if you acknowledge its power over you and the impact it has on you, and recognize that as the anniversary passes, the pain associated with the memory will diminish.

January and February—The Dark Days

Now the time you have been planning for has arrived—the two worst months of the year. But if your plans are in place and if you handle them—and yourself—correctly, you should be able to avoid the darkest times of the spirit. I hope that you can find the opportunity to travel toward the sun, even if only for a short time. If you do not, you will need to soldier, but there are many things you can do to help yourself through these days. Some of these I have already outlined in the previous chapters, though I will summarize them here again. Other strategies can be learned by examining the lives of those who have overcome their condition to some extent and have managed to find joy in this darkest of seasons. Meanwhile, though, the dark days are upon you. Look through the following checklist and see which of the guidelines you have already incorporated into your life and which may yet be worth trying:

▶ **Get more light in any safe way you can:**
  - Use your dawn simulator.
  - Keep the shutters in your bedroom open.
  - Go outdoors whenever you can while the sun is shining.
  - Drive around in your car when the sun is out.
  - Enjoy the sunlight reflected off snow.
  - Use your light box regularly.
  - Brighten up your home.
  - Spend time in the brightest room.

▶ **Minimize your stress:**
  - Don't undertake unnecessary chores.
  - Delay that which can be delayed.
  - Meditate.
  - Don't allow guilt to prevent you from saying no to new burdens and commitments.

▶ Explain to others what is going on and tell them how they can help make life easier for you.
▶ Exercise as much as you can.
▶ If you are not on medications and are still laboring under the burden of winter, discuss with your doctor the possibility of starting them.
▶ If you are on medications that do not seem to be doing their job, discuss with your doctor the possibility of modifying your medication regimen.
▶ Keep a journal.
▶ Find out what brings you pleasure and do more of it.
▶ Find out what brings you displeasure and do less of it.
▶ Buy some forced bulbs and watch them grow and bloom in these dark months, reminders that spring is not so far away—what one of my patients called "tulip therapy." I find amaryllis plants especially encouraging because their rapid growth dramatizes

the passage of time, while their brilliant flowers foreshadow the return of the sun.

- Accept that winter may never feel as good as the other seasons, no matter how hard you try to cope with it.
- Accept the downtime, the quiet of this dormant season.
- Wait for spring—it will arrive. It always does.

March and April—Spring

At the end of winter there is a season
in which we are daily expecting spring
and finally a day when it arrives.
A flock of geese . . .
now in the dark flying low over the pond . . .
I stood at my door and could hear their wings.
—HENRY DAVID THOREAU

Spring comes in different ways in different places, and we each have our own way of feeling this crucial transition from the season of darkness to the season of light. For most people with SAD, the arrival of spring is met with exhilaration. It is like water to a parched desert wanderer, or food to a starving man. It is an overwhelming relief. But there are some who experience pain in this transition and feel left out of the general carnival spirit that everyone around them appears to be celebrating. If you are such a person, pay attention to how you are feeling at this transition time, recognizing that not everyone experiences spring in the same way.

For those who experience the more usual resurgence of energy, spring is a good time to pick up tasks left undone through the winter. It is no coincidence that spring cleaning occurs in spring. But be sure to enjoy the season; you have waited for it and labored long and hard through the winter to get here.

When spring arrives, don't pack away your lights too quickly—it can be a volatile season.

Be sure not to pack away your lights, your winter ways, and winter paraphernalia too quickly. Spring is a volatile time that can make your mood whiz forward to its summer state or pull you right back into the gloom of winter, depending on the weather. So keep your eyes on the skies—and take action according to what you see there.

"How Can I Help?"

ADVICE FOR FAMILY AND FRIENDS

> ▶ What can I do to help a person with SAD?
>
> ▶ How much should I do to fill in when the person has low energy and motivation?
>
> Other people can be a terrific source of comfort and support to someone with SAD. If you are a relative or friend of a seasonal patient, the following information should help you fill that role.

Things to Do

1. *Understand the problem.* Recognize that the seasonal mood problem is a real affliction. This may be hard to appreciate, especially for people who have never themselves been depressed. More mildly afflicted friends and relatives also have a hard time understanding how bad people with SAD can actually feel. It is important to realize that severity makes a big difference. I would encourage friends and relatives of the seasonal person to read some of the stories in the earlier part of this book to gain insight into how disabling the problem can be.

It can be helpful to think of SAD as similar, in certain critical ways, to a physical illness. We do not know what the underlying abnormality is in SAD, but it presumably resides somewhere in the brain, where some chemical processes do not function normally, resulting in all the symptoms of the condition. Somehow, light entering the eyes plays an important role in these key chemical processes. During the short, dark days of winter, when there is not enough light in the environment, the brain-chemical abnormalities become manifest in the form of SAD symptoms. Bright light reverses the symptoms, presumably by correcting the underlying abnormalities. As a diabetic needs insulin shots and may need encouragement to go along with the program, your friend or relative with SAD needs extra light and can benefit tremendously from your support. You can help, for example, by keeping your friend or relative company while he or she is sitting in front of the lights.

Once you understand the mood and energy problems of SAD, you will be able to handle them better. If your spouse falls behind in paying the bills or carrying out various chores when winter arrives, it will be much easier for you to put up with the resulting inconvenience once you understand that you are probably dealing with SAD rather than laziness. If you want to find

Recognizing that inertia is probably a result of SAD can help you deal with any inconvenience caused by it.

out more about the condition and its treatments, you may find parts of this book helpful.

2. *Just be there.* Don't feel you have to do anything specific. Your undemanding presence and company will be experienced as soothing and helpful. Despite any appearance of being withdrawn and unfriendly, the seasonal person will often appreciate having company. As one man I know puts it, "I want my friends to tolerate me sitting solemnly in a corner reading a magazine. I like people to be around but not asking very much of me, because I don't have very much to give." A woman echoes this need for understanding, noting that when you are depressed, "you get into a place where it's hard for a person to relate to you unless he really cares about you, has known you for a while, and understands your seasonality." She recognizes that "people don't like their friends to change. It's hard for the people you live with," but she asks her friends not to expect her to be "bubbly and full of myself like I am in the summer . . . just accept me the way I am."

3. *Encourage the seasonal person.* Remind him that this is a passing phase, that he has not always felt this way, and that he can and

will feel better again. A person who is lethargic and uninspired during the depths of the winter may be kind, friendly, charming, or witty at other times of the year. Remind him about the good times. When you're depressed, it's easy to forget that they ever happened, as well as forgetting everything you have ever learned about depression. At such a time a friend or relative who understands what is happening can help tremendously simply by saying "Hey, you're forgetting, this is your winter problem. It will pass."

4. *Help with simple things.* Sometimes even shopping or laundry can feel like a huge chore to the depressed person. Offers by friends and family to help out with these will generally be greatly appreciated. One family had a system of rotating household chores weekly, some of which were easier and others more difficult. During the winter, the children understood that their mother was not able to tackle the more difficult chores, and they all agreed that she should be exempt from bathroom duty during those months.

The best way to find out what help is needed is to ask. Even the smallest things will be remembered and rewarded by a deepening and strengthening of your relationship.

HOW CAN YOU HELP?

- Can you go to the grocery store for a friend?
- Fix breakfast for your husband?
- Help your wife get the kids off to school while she sits in front of her lights?
- Sit and talk to a friend or loved one while he does the laundry or pays the bills?
- Help the seasonal person with the difficult task of waking up in the morning?

5. *Try to understand the seasonal person when he or she is in the hypomanic phase.* Sometimes it's difficult to understand the high side of SAD as well. Someone who has been hibernating all winter and suddenly springs into action with more energy than anyone else may be hard to

take. As one woman puts it, "I think it's easier to love someone who's down and depressed and hurting in some way. But please remember to love her when she's happy and successful as well." It may also be helpful to point out *tactfully* that the seasonal person is going a bit fast for you and most other people and that it may be useful to get some help slowing down a bit. Encourage your friend or relative to avoid being exposed to too much bright light. Sleeping with the bedroom shades down or wearing dark glasses during daylight hours may help people slow down at such times if they are too wired.

> A seasonal person who is showing poor judgment, impulsiveness, or sleeplessness should be encouraged (or taken) to see his or her psychiatrist.

When people are a bit high, they can become argumentative. The friend or relative exposed to such querulousness would do well to choose carefully what issues to bring up. The husband of one of my seasonal patients has learned the value of this strategy over the years, and avoids confronting his wife on minor issues. As he says, "If we have a conflict, it's going to be over something worthwhile."

Things to Avoid

1. *Don't judge and criticize.* The seasonal person is already feeling bad about not functioning up to her normal standards and letting friends and family down. Very often she is her own harshest critic, measuring her own actions and finding them wanting. To have these criticisms confirmed by someone she loves and respects can be extremely painful, may further undermine her self-esteem, and could enhance feelings of depression and worthlessness. A tendency to judge and criticize the seasonal person is very understandable, but it stems from a fundamental misconception that the seasonal person is willfully declining to do certain things or is being self-indulgent and weak-willed and is giving in to passing moods.

It may be helpful for you to think back to some time when you were feeling weak, tired, or out of sorts, perhaps due to a physical condition such as an infection or operation. Imagine how it would have felt to be criticized at such a time for not meeting your obligations with sufficient energy or enthusiasm. One young man who has been in and out of seasonal depressions for the past several years still finds it difficult to convince his friends that he has been suffering from an illness. They continue to regard his months of withdrawal and impaired functioning as a character disturbance or failure of will. As a result, he is beginning to reevaluate these friendships.

2. *Don't take the seasonal person's withdrawal personally.* You should not assume that he or she is mad at you or uninterested in being friends with you. One patient thinks back on friends who have called her during her down times and said, "Well, I've called you the last three times. Do you really want to be friends anymore?" She observes, "That kind of situation seems to pop up all the time in the winter. I understand that other people need certain things from a friendship, but it comes at a time when even getting up to answer the phone is a major effort: Who is it going to be? What do I have to talk about now? The best kind of friend is someone who is willing to keep calling you and to keep saying 'Do you feel like doing anything?' I'm not saying that friends should baby you, nor do they have to sit there and hold your hand. It's very simple: Just accept someone who is in a different place." The same person recalls hurtful conversations with friends who have not understood her difficulty. "They say, 'Oh, yeah, here you go again,' and it's sort of mocking. They just don't understand."

3. *Don't assume that it is your responsibility to make the seasonal person feel fine.* It's not likely to work, and you will probably end up feeling frustrated and irritated at your failure. When you feel responsible for bringing a person out of a depression and you have failed to do so, you are likely to feel angry. You have sunk so much energy into trying to reverse the situation that you may be inclined to see the depressed person as having caused you to fail. You will then be more likely to blame him for making you feel that way. You might attribute your "failure" to a willful attempt on his part to resist all help and, in your anger, feel inclined to say that if he is not willing to accept your helping hand, he deserves to remain in a slump. As I have noted already, anger tends to get turned on the depressed person just when he feels least capable of coping with even the most ordinary things in life, let alone problems with a dear friend or relative. The key to not getting angry is understanding the problem and not feeling responsible for fixing it. But do remember that simple things, such as being there for your friend or family member, can make an enormous difference.

Part III

Celebrating the Seasons

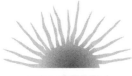

FOURTEEN

A Brief History of Seasonal Time

▶ How have the changing seasons taught us about time itself?

▶ What can we learn today from the cyclical nature of the seasons?

▶ What can the seasons do for us besides give us light and then take it away?

So far, I have discussed the discomfort and disability the seasons can cause and have considered light largely as a medication. These factors, however, account for only a small part of the effect that light and the seasons have on the mind. The seasons provided an impetus for the development of our solar calendar and helped us come to terms, both intellectually and emotionally, with the passing of time. The fluxes in mood, energy, and vitality that may be experienced with the changing seasons have infused many people with creative energy that has been the source of many of their finest achievements. These internal changes, coinciding as they do with those in the natural world, have inspired artists and writers to express, visually in words, the shifting beauty of their landscape. In this chapter and those that follow, let us consider how the seasons have opened our minds to seeing our world in new and interesting ways.

*A*lthough the solar calendar may seem commonplace to us, since we use it on a daily basis, our earliest measure of time was based on the more obvious monthly cycle of the moon. The calendar helped ancient civilizations predict the changing seasons and decide when to plant their crops. A major problem with the lunar year, which consisted of 12 months, was that it fell short of the 365-day solar year by several days. As a result, the lunar year gradually shifted out of phase with the seasons. In an attempt to correct these shifts, certain societies inserted extra months at intervals into their lunar calendar.

The Solar Calendar: The Key to Measuring Time

The Egyptians have been given credit for developing the solar calendar. They used their ability to predict where the sun would fall on a given day to illuminate their obelisks and add drama to their religious festivals. Many societies have since used the similar principle of knowing where a slab of light or shadow would fall on a particular day—for example, the winter or summer solstice—to enhance their sense of awe over a mysterious, yet predictable, universe. The solar calendar—as measured, for example, by the sundial—worked well, and still does, in predicting the changing seasons.

The problem of anticipating seasonal changes in the world around us has not been an exclusively human one. For many animals, especially those that live at some distance from the equator, it is crucial to be able to anticipate when it will be cold or hot, when food will be scarce or plentiful, and when to mate, migrate, or hibernate. As described in Chapter 4, from the lowly *Gonyaulax* alga that causes red tides to domestic animals such as sheep and horses, every organism must be able to anticipate the seasons so as to make the appropriate adaptive changes. To time such events correctly, all these animals have evolved complex physiological programs that depend for their accurate timing on information from the physical world. The environmental time cue of greatest importance across a multitude of species, including perhaps humans, is the length of the day, which is a function of the solar year. Thus our solar calendar and the calendar of our biological responses both follow the annual course of the sun across the sky. The solar calendar, the product of human intellect, and the seasonal patterns of biology, shaped over hundreds of thousands of years by the forces of evolution, have both used the sun and the seasons as the most dependable and meaningful markers for charting time over long periods.

Cyclical Time: Wiping the Slate Clean Every Year

Quite apart from the practical need to measure time, humans have also had to deal with the emotional impact of its passing. Over the course of time, we receive the gifts of life, health, youth, and children, and the rewards of our labors; yet in time we lose them all. We are subject to aging, disease, the destructive forces of our fellow human beings, and finally, death. How do we come to terms with all these losses, as well as with the burden of the errors we have made?

These are age-old problems, and ancient humans found a novel solution to them: Simply abolish time. Wipe it out and start all over again. Thus, in ancient times, at the end of each year, people engaged in cleansing rituals, purifying themselves of the dirt and sin they had accumulated over the previous year. They could then enter the new year fresh and clean. All manner of complex rituals were developed. For example, sins would be transferred to a goat, and the animal would be driven out of the area—the proverbial scapegoat. Not only were one's sins abolished, but the slate of time was itself wiped clean. Ancient humans lacked a sense that one year led to the next—a concept of time that has been termed *linear* or *historical.* Instead, they believed in cyclical time, "the myth of the eternal return," which happens to be the title of a fascinating book on the subject by Mircea Eliade.

Around the time of the winter solstice, it was traditional to extinguish and rekindle fire. Even in modern times, the festivals that take place around the time of the winter solstice are celebrated with lights: the colored ones on Christmas trees and the candles on a Hanukkah menorah. In some cultures, the winter solstice coincides with the new year, and the extinguishing and rekindling of fire could also be regarded as symbolizing the obliteration of time past and the start of new time. Alternatively, such activities might be viewed as a celebration of (or prayer for) the return of the sun's light following the winter solstice. The use of light in these rituals may also serve to lift our spirits during the darkest days of the year.

Cyclical time was common in many ancient societies. The Greeks conceived of history as cyclical and developed the idea of a "Great Year" many thousands of solar years in length. The Great Year, which they believed corresponded to the rotation of the heavens, had a Great Summer, when planetary forces would combine to destroy the earth by fire, and a Great Winter, when the world would be overwhelmed by water. The Indians had a similar concept of a cosmic cycle, called a *Mahayuga*, which was thought to last four million years.

Linear Time: A Mixed Blessing

It seems likely that the obvious seasonal changes in the world around us and our internal changes in mood and behavior, together perhaps with the wish to abolish the past, all contributed to the development of a cyclical sense of time. In the last few centuries, however, a linear or historical one has prevailed. This sense of time is familiar to every schoolchild who has had to construct a dateline showing how certain events occurred over the years. An integral part of this concept is that these events took place in a certain sequence and that, in certain critical ways, the clock or calendar cannot be turned back. Thus, World War II took place in part because of unresolved issues from World War I. Dropping the atom bombs on Japan put an end to World War II, an event that could not have happened 4 years earlier, since the atom bomb had not yet been invented. The dropping of the bomb ushered in an age in which nuclear warfare is an ever-present possibility. That has changed the nature of war and the whole way we view our world. Thus, nowadays, even schoolchildren become thoroughly familiar with the concept of linear or historical time that moves in one direction only.

The Jews have been credited with the development of the sense of linear time. Calamities that beset the children of Israel were interpreted by the prophets as the result of the wrath of God, proof that the people needed to reform their ways. The prophets thus forced the people to turn away from a purely cyclical and ever-renewing sense of time and face the consequences of their actions. This concept was continued in

Christianity, which sees time as a straight line that traces the course of humanity from its creation through Redemption to the present. The Chinese, in their descriptions of successive dynasties, have been credited with independently coming up with a linear sense of time, and such a sense was surely present in the mind of the 13th-century Japanese sage Dogen, who observed, "Time flies more swiftly than an arrow and life is more transient than the dew. We cannot call back a single day that has passed."

> A linear sense of time helps us learn from history and pursue progress, but ignoring the cyclical aspect of time may blind us to how the cycles of seasons affect us—as in SAD.

According to Eliade, the conflict between the two different perceptions of time—cyclical and linear—continued into the 17th century, after which the latter view gained ascendance. This was in keeping with the development of science, the theory of evolution, and the idea of human progress, all of which were believed to proceed in a linear way. Despite this linear trend, both Jews and Christians have continued to celebrate cyclical time in the form of seasonal rituals and festivals. There was a renewal of interest in cyclical time in the 20th century. Historians such as Oswald Spengler and Arnold Toynbee considered the problems of periodicity in history. The works of two important modern writers, T. S. Eliot and James Joyce, are, in Eliade's view, "saturated with nostalgia for the myth of eternal repetition and . . . the abolition of time."

One of the reasons it took modern scientists so long to recognize SAD might have been the ascendance of linear over cyclical time. According to a linear way of thinking, a psychiatrist might consider, for example, a patient with three episodes of winter depression as follows:

Three years ago, in October, she broke up with her boyfriend and became depressed for several months. By April, she recovered, moved, and found a new job. She was not able to function for long in this position, however, became depressed, and lost the job in December. The next March, she entered into a new relationship, which seemed to lift her spirits. She was well until about a month ago (October), when her relationship difficulties resurfaced, and she has since become markedly lethargic, withdrawn, and depressed.

If the same psychiatrist paid attention to the cyclical nature of time as well, he might see that the patient's problems started at the same time every year and receded at the same time every year—and suggest the obvious diagnosis, SAD.

In recent decades, we have once again become interested in cyclicity in the form of biological rhythms. It was this developing interest that served as a major precursor to the recognition and description of SAD. And yet we often still have trouble recognizing the effects of the seasons upon us—just like the people of Tromsø, Norway, who are described in the next chapter.

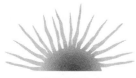

FIFTEEN

Polar Tales

The days are growing rapidly shorter and the nights,
only too noticeably longer. . . . It is this discouraging
veil of blackness, falling over the sparkling whiteness
of earlier nights, which sends a vein of despair running
through our souls.

—FREDERICK COOK, *Through the First Antarctic Night*

- What can the seasonal experiences of those living in the northernmost countries tell us?

- Do they adapt to the extremes of light and darkness or suffer more from SAD than countries closer to the equator?

- Why haven't their experiences led the way in SAD research?

I have frequently been asked, "Have they studied SAD in Scandinavia? Don't they get a lot of it over there?" Since our work at the NIMH first appeared, Scandinavian research groups have done considerable work on the subject. Before then, however, there was little or nothing about it in Scandinavian medical literature. Given the degree of light deprivation so far north, that was surprising. Were Scandinavians particularly resistant to the problems of SAD? Had their researchers simply overlooked its importance? One Swedish psychiatrist provided a witty answer: "Either everyone there has SAD," he replied, "or no one does."

Since then, thanks to studies by several Scandinavian researchers, it has become apparent that approximately one in three adults in the far north is affected adversely by the winter season. Icelanders might be an exception, possibly protected biologically against the dark days, as mentioned in Chapter 4. Nevertheless, Andrés Magnusson, a psychiatrist from Iceland, notes that "everyone seems to have some relative who takes to bed for the whole winter." Cases that sound like SAD can also be found, according to Magnusson, in Icelandic myths. Seasonal changes in behavior are reportedly rife in the population as a whole; they are so widespread in the far North, according to some observers, that most people just take them for granted. This may be why they did not attract the attention of the medical community until reports started appearing from other parts of the world.

In fact, some of the best descriptions of the behavioral effects of circumpolar winters come from outsiders. Frederick Cook, for example, who went on a 19th-century expedition to Antarctica as ship's doctor to the *Belgica*, described how the crew suffered from isolation and harsh weather while trapped in the ice during the Antarctic winter. The 68 consecutive days of darkness appeared to affect the men badly, and, according to Cook, they "gradually . . . became affected, body and soul, with languor." He described other psychiatric problems among the crew, concluding, "The root cause of these disasters was the lack of the sun." He found that treating his men with direct exposure to an open fire seemed to help them, perhaps more because of the light than the heat.

Cook also provided us with a description of the seasonal rhythms of sexual drive among the Eskimos: "The passions of these people are periodical, and their courtship is usually carried on soon after the return of the sun; in fact, at this time, they almost tremble from the intensity of their passions and for several weeks most of their time is taken up in gratifying them."

Such shifts in sex drive, with a surge of interest in the spring, continuing into the summer, almost certainly affect people living at lower latitudes, though to a lesser degree. Many societies have created spring rituals that incorporate elements of sexuality or fertility, which coincide with the burgeoning of nature outside and rising sexual passions within.

An excellent description of the psychological effects of the dark days on the people of Tromsø in northern Norway was provided by Joseph Wechsberg, who wrote an article in *The New Yorker* in 1972 called "Mørketiden," which means, "murky times." Tromsø, which lies 215 miles north of the Arctic Circle, has 59 sunless days during the winter. Wechsberg observed that "the people talked a lot about mørketiden, and at the same time protested that they were not affected by it." He reported that people felt tired, had difficulty getting up in the morning and accomplishing their work, and suffered from disturbed sleep, low energy level, and actual depression. In other words, many of these people complained of the symptoms of SAD. One man he interviewed even observed that the depression seemed to be a problem particularly among women.

Wechsberg described an opposite pattern of behavior in the summer. People rarely seemed to feel tired and often did not feel like going to bed.

> *Inhabitants of northern Norway talked a lot about their sunless 2 months every year but insisted the lack of light didn't bother them.*

They were active at all hours of the night. There was widespread celebration as people headed for the country to "fish, hunt, have fun." As a result, it was difficult to get any work done.

Wechsberg observed that in winter the people of Tromsø kept their indoor lights on constantly during the day. One woman reported missing the sun so much that she gravitated toward the window. The return of the sun after 59 dark days was celebrated as *soldag*, or sun day. Children were sent home early from school that day, and all work stopped by noon. The first rays were greeted with tears, prayers, and special wishes. Some people, unwilling to wait for this day, flew to southern Norway to see the sun.

Since Wechsberg's article, the effects of the seasons on mood and behavior have been studied in Tromsø and elsewhere in Scandinavia. I have since visited Tromsø twice myself, both in the summer and in the winter. In the summer, looking out of the window of my hotel across the bay, I could not tell whether it was day or night. Traffic crossed the bridge at all hours of the 24-hour day, people walked about in the streets, and human behavior provided no clue as to the time of day. I felt euphoric at first and later unpleasantly revved up and exhausted, and sleep would not have been possible had I not pulled down the blackout shades installed specifically for that purpose. In the town there was merriment well into the early hours of the morning.

How different the town looked in winter. The streets were covered in snow under the dark purple-black cover of the sky. There was a silver rim on the horizon, a reflection off the clouds of the sun shining somewhere far away, south of the Arctic Circle. Tramping through the snow at night, I felt a peaceful stillness in the crisp air, while overhead the northern lights were faintly visible, like a diaphanous curtain waving gently in an impalpable breeze. Small wonder that the natives of the North believed these mysterious lights were torches to guide the spirits of the dead to the world beyond.

Many people diagnosed with SAD are amazed to think that they missed the pattern for so many years. I wonder whether people living in the far north might have a similar reaction.

> *Were you so used to the negative effects of the seasons that you took them for granted for years before recognizing that you had a right to feel better?*

Research indicating that seasonal difficulties are common in Tromsø has not been universally appreciated. Many have commented that the story is greatly overblown and that a fuss is being made of nothing. Perhaps the stoicism of the North prevents many of these people from acknowledging their difficulties. The dramatic seasons have always been part of their lives, and they may regard them as a law of nature, immutable and therefore to be accepted without complaint. In contrast, perhaps my own upbringing in a climate where the seasons were mild enabled me to recognize that the dramatic seasonal changes in North America were not a necessary part of life. As in Edgar Allan Poe's story of the purloined letter, sometimes that which is right under one's nose is most difficult to observe.

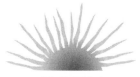

SIXTEEN

Creating with the Seasons

Great Wits are sure to Madness near ally'd,
And thin Partitions do their Bounds divide.
—JOHN DRYDEN

> ‣ Have great artists of the past suffered from psychiatric disturbances?
>
> ‣ If so, what forms have these disturbances taken?
>
> ‣ Where do seasonal responses fit into this picture, if at all?
>
> ‣ Does sensitivity to light—a cardinal feature of people with SAD—seem to go along with sensitivity to our exterior and interior worlds?
>
> The association between genius and insanity is ingrained in our culture. We are told about the "thin line" that exists between the brilliant artist and the madman. Is there any truth to this assertion? Can those with SAD learn anything beneficial from such a connection if it in fact exists? This chapter explores these fascinating questions.

The Link among Mood Disorders, Creativity, and the Seasons

The concept that genius and madness are somehow connected goes back at least to the time of Aristotle, who observed that "no great genius was without a mixture of insanity." He added, "Those who have become eminent in philosophy, politics, poetry, and the arts have all had tendencies toward melancholia." The Roman playwright Seneca echoed this view, noting that "the mind cannot attain anything lofty so long as it is sane." For centuries this belief persisted, and melancholia was somehow endowed with cultural value. Genius was regarded as a hereditary trait transmitted in families, along with mental illness.

It is only in our century, however, that the subject has been a matter of serious study. Nancy Andreasen was the first researcher to study the relationship between creativity and mental illness using modern psychiatric diagnoses. She interviewed 30 creative writers at the prestigious Iowa Writers' Workshop about their own backgrounds and those of their close relatives and compared their responses with those of 30 control subjects. She found a substantially higher rate of mental illness among the writers and their family members. She had approached the study with the belief that there would be an association between schizophrenia and creativity. To her surprise, it was not schizophrenia but disorders of mood regulation—especially those involving a tendency to mania or hypomania, in addition to depression—that distinguished the writers from the control group. She concluded that the traits of creativity and mood disturbance appeared to run together in families and might be genetically mediated.

Later, Kay Redfield Jamison studied a group of eminent British writers and artists for evidence of psychiatric illness, seasonal variations in mood and productivity, and the perceived role of intense moods in their creative processes. She selected these artists and writers on the basis of objective acclaim, in the form of prestigious prizes and other types of acknowledgment. She interviewed them extensively and found very high rates of mood disorders in the group. Over one-third had been treated for mood problems, the great majority with medications or hospitalization. Poets were most likely to require medication for depression and were the only group to require treatment for mania.

Playwrights had the highest total rate of treatment for mood disorders, but a high percentage of this group had been treated with psychotherapy alone. Exceptional among the writers in regard to their mood stability were biographers, who reported no history of mood swings or elated states. Although these writers were as outstanding as the others, in terms of their objective achievements, they were perhaps a less creative group.

Almost all subjects—with the exception of the biographers—reported having had intense, highly productive, and creative periods. Most of these lasted between 1 and 4 weeks. These episodes were marked by "increased enthusiasm, energy, self-confidence, speed of mental association, fluency of thoughts, elevated mood, and a strong sense of well-being." They sound very much like hypomanic episodes, without the behavioral disturbance that term implies. Ninety percent of Jamison's group reported that very intense moods and feelings were either integral to or necessary for the development and execution of their work.

Investigating the association among seasons, mood, and productivity, Jamison found a strong seasonal pattern of mood changes among artists and writers, with highest mood scores in the summer and lowest in the winter. Peak periods of productivity, while also seasonal, occurred in the spring and the fall. It seemed that as mood increased from spring to summer, productivity declined to some extent, picking up again in the fall. Those who had been treated for mood disorders had a sharper decline of productivity in the summer than the other subjects.

> Artists with seasonal mood changes may be most productive in spring and fall rather than summer, because in summer they are either too scattered or just having too much fun to work. Can you take advantage of the two seasons—spring and fall—when you need to be your most creative?

A few possible explanations for this drop-off in creativity in the summer—as mood continues to improve—come to mind. When people are too euphoric, they are often not best able to produce. Their thoughts may race too quickly, and their focus may be scattered. There is a tendency to start many tasks but not to follow through—distractibility is a problem. Those subjects in Jamison's study who had been treated for mood disorders might have experienced more marked highs during the summer, with greater associated difficulties in focusing and carrying out tasks. Another possibility is that the artist might not wish to be creative during the summer. One writer I know with SAD said that she has so much fun in the summer that she doesn't want to spend her golden, sunny days bashing away at a computer.

The Lifetime Creativity Scale was developed by Ruth Richards and Dennis Kinney of Harvard University as a means of measuring creativity. The advantage of this scale is that it can be used to measure creativity in anyone, not just in those of exceptional talent. By means of the scale, these researchers were able to show a higher rate of creativity than expected among people with bipolar disorder, but even greater creativity scores among their relatives—those with milder mood swings or no clear-cut mood swings at all. The heightened level of creativity found in relatives of people with bipolar disorder may explain why the illness has been transmitted so successfully from generation to generation. People who carry bipolar genes may be at an advantage to survive and reproduce by virtue of their creative talents. People with bipolar tendencies and their relatives seem more likely to take risks, such as emigrating, which may be highly adaptive in crisis situations.

All these studies suggest that Aristotle had a point when he linked mood disturbance and creativity. It seems as though the *most* creative people are those with milder forms of mood disturbance, which is in keeping with my clinical experience. Severe depressions or wild manias are not conducive to productivity. The opposite is true for mild depressions (or dysthymia) alternating with hypomanic episodes. During hypomanic periods, thoughts and associations flow rapidly, energy and confidence levels are high, the need for sleep is reduced, and ideas are more readily generated and pursued. Later, during dysthymic periods, these ideas can be evaluated critically. Ideas that are too grandiose or unlikely to succeed can be discarded, and those

> *Mild forms of mood disturbance—such as often occur in SAD—are most likely to be conducive to creativity, whereas severe depression and mania interfere with productivity.*

that look most promising in the more sober light of dysthymia can be retained and developed. Mild depressions may be conducive to the drudgery that is required for any creative venture—the daily plodding necessary to execute any grand scheme.

The seasonal person will easily recognize this pattern of mood swings and its relationship to creativity, for the depressions of SAD are often relatively mild in severity, the hypomania restrained and productive. As we now know, the mood changes in people with SAD are often driven by the amount of ambient daylight. Many creative artists have recognized the connection between changes in environmental light and their mood and productivity. The following section describes some famous creative people who suffered from mood disorders—especially those in whom there is evidence of strong seasonality or light sensitivity.

Moody and Famous: Sensitive to Seasons and Light

There's a certain Slant of light,
Winter Afternoons—
That oppresses, like the Heft
Of Cathedral Tunes–
    —EMILY DICKINSON

The list of famous people with mood disturbances is impressive. Although there was no psychiatrist with a modern diagnostic handbook around to record the mental status of most of the people in this section, abundant evidence for mood disorders exists in most cases. It is not my purpose here to be comprehensive, only to select some illustrative examples of famous creative people with mood disorders. Among artists we have Michelangelo, Albrecht Dürer, and Vincent van Gogh; composers include George Frideric Handel, Gustav Mahler, and Robert Schumann; writers include John Milton, Edgar Allan Poe, Ernest Hemingway, and Virginia Woolf; politicians include Abraham Lincoln and Winston Churchill, who referred to his depressions as his "black dog." Sir Isaac Newton was perhaps the most eminent scientist to have suffered from bipolar disorder (manic–depression).

How many of these people were strongly seasonal in their mood swings or sensitive to changes in environmental light is hard to say with clinical certainty, especially since SAD as a distinct entity was first described long after all of these artists were deceased. Statistically, it is highly likely that many of these people were seasonal. Figures for the rate of SAD among people with recurrent depression range from one in six to one in three. Highly creative people with mood disorders are more likely to have SAD than other forms of mood disorder, most of which are more disruptive to productivity. Beyond such general statistical information, however, we do have specific clues about seasonality and light sensitivity in several cases.

Among writers, Emily Dickinson is a likely candidate for a diagnosis of SAD. Not only did she write about the slant of light on winter afternoons, but she declared that she could not "meet the Spring unmoved," and, on summer days, described herself as an "inebriate of air" and "debauchee of dew." T. S. Eliot might be another patient for this distinguished clinic. His poetry sparkles with references to light. We learn that Eliot was instructed by his doctors to go south each winter. Could that have been to treat his SAD? We can only speculate. Milton is reputed to have suffered from summer SAD and, according to his biographer, was able to work on *Paradise Lost* during only half the year, between autumn and spring.

Another writer with a light-sensitive mood disorder was Guy de Maupassant. Toward the end of his life he attempted suicide and went on to die in an asylum. The following extract is from a story called "Who Knows?" in which the narrator, who ends up in an asylum, recalls how he went to Italy, where the sunlight made him feel good. After that, he recounts,

> I returned to France via Marseilles, and in spite of the gaiety of Provence, the diminished intensity of sunlight depressed me. On my return to the Continent, I had the odd feeling of a patient who thinks he is cured but who is warned by a dull pain that the source of illness has not been eradicated.

Was de Maupassant seasonal? It seems like a fair bet.

Among musicians, Handel and Mahler were most clearly seasonal. Both, we are told, did most of their creative work during the summer months. One of the most prodigiously rapid feats of composition was Handel's *Messiah*, which he completed in 23 days, between late August and mid-September. Mahler, who called himself the "summer composer," was fortunately an avid letter writer. His seasonal mood changes are apparent in his letters. Consider the following letter, written in summer.

> To Joseph Steiner, Puzsta-Batta, June 19, 1879
>
> Dear Steiner,
>
> Now for the third day I return to you, and today I do so in order to take leave of you in merry mood. It is the story of my life that is recorded in these pages. What a strange destiny, sweeping me along on the waves of my yearning, now hurling me this way and that in the gale, now wafting me along merrily in smiling sunshine. What I fear is that in such a gale I shall someday be shattered against a reef—such as my keel has often grazed!
>
> It is six o'clock in the morning! I have been out on the heath, sitting with Fárkas the shepherd, listening to the sound of his shawm. Ah, how mournful it sounded, and yet how full of rapturous delight—that folk-tune he played! Ah, Steiner! You are still asleep in your bed, and I have already seen the dew on the grasses. I am now so serenely gay and the tranquil happiness all around me is tiptoeing into my heart, too, as the sun of early spring lights up the wintry fields. Is spring awakening now in my own breast?! And while this mood prevails, let me take leave of you, my faithful friend!

Contrast that with a winter postcard sent to Friedrich Löhr, dated January 20, 1883.

> Dear Fritz,
>
> Simply cannot find time to write to you properly. Sending the stuff soon. My address is: . . . Am extremely depressed.
>
> Very best wishes to you and your family,
>
> Yours,
>
> Gustav

But two years later, in spring, Mahler wrote to the same friend:

My dear Fritz,

My windows are open and the sunny, fragrant spring is gazing in upon me, everywhere endless peace and repose. In this fair hour that is granted me I will be together with you. . . .
    With the coming of spring all has grown mild in me again. From my window I have a view across the city to the mountains and woods, and the kindly Fulda wends its amiable way between; whenever the sun casts its colored lights within, as now, well, you know how everything in one relaxes. That is the mood I am in today, sitting at my desk by the window, from time to time casting a peaceful glance out upon this scene of carefree calm.

These are just a few of the many letters suggesting that Mahler suffered from SAD.

Painters and sculptors are more difficult to diagnose in retrospect than writers, but Jamison's work would suggest that they are as susceptible to mood disturbances. Artists, perhaps more than any other group, have struggled to portray light. In fact, the works of some can be instantly recognized by the distinctive quality of the light they portray: Turner's swirls of light; Rembrandt's splashes of chiaroscuro, illuminating the pensive faces of his models; and, of course, the dazzling colors of Vincent van Gogh.

Could the genes for creativity and mood disorders be transmitted together? If so, would it be better to keep those genes and deal with the mood swings—like those of SAD—rather than to modify them and possibly disrupt creativity in the process? That is the sort of question we might have to confront one of these days when we are able to tinker with our genomes.

Of these three painters, the only one with a clear history of a mood disorder is van Gogh. It seems very likely that he suffered from bipolar disorder, although his clinical picture was complicated by intoxication with absinthe, the French liquor that at that time had a toxic ingredient in it. Van Gogh's intimate understanding of depression is apparent in his famous sketches, *Sorrow* and *The Old Man in Sorrow*. In contrast to these sad figures is *The Reaper*, a young man striding boldly across a field with a huge, luminous sun shining in the background. Van Gogh's groundbreaking use of light and color might make one suspect that he was extremely sensitive to light, and indeed, his letters to his beloved brother Theo appear to bear this out. They are suffused with feelings of sadness and joy and his sensitivity to the weather, and to light and darkness in particular. Here are a few selections (reprinted from Irving Stone's *Dear Theo*):

[Autumn in Drenthe, 1883]

When I look around me, everything seems too miserable, too insufficient, too dilapidated. We are having gloomy days of rain now, and when I come to the corner of the garret where I have settled down, it is curiously melancholy there; through one single glass pane the light falls on an empty colour box, on a bundle of brushes the hair of which is quite worn down. It is so strangely melancholy that it has, luckily, almost a comical aspect—enough not to make one cry over it. As long as the weather was fine I did not mind my troubles, because I saw so many beautiful things; but with this rainy weather, which we must expect to continue for months, I see more clearly how I have got stuck here, and how handicapped I am.

[Winter in Nuenen, 1883]

Hardly ever have I begun a year of gloomier aspect, or in a gloomier mood. It is dreary outside; the fields are a mass of lumps of black earth and some snow, with days mostly of mist and mire. . . . This is what I see in passing, and it is quite in harmony with the interiors, very gloomy these dark winter days.

[Spring in The Hague, 1892]

Spring is coming fast here. We have had a few real spring days; last Monday, for instance, which I enjoyed very much. I think the poor people and the painters have in common this feeling for the weather and the change of the seasons.

In February 1888, Vincent van Gogh left Paris for Arles, in the south of France, at least in part to escape the darkness of the North and seek out the brilliant and dazzling light of Provence. In van Gogh's own words,

I came to the south for a thousand reasons. I wanted to see a different light, I believed that by looking at nature under a bright sky one might gain a truer idea of the Japanese way of feeling and drawing. Finally, I wanted to see this stronger sun . . . because I felt that the colors of the spectrum are misted over in the north.

Here is a description to his brother Theo, written from Arles in the summer of 1888:

The loneliness has not worried me, because I have found the brighter sun and its effect on nature so absorbing. . . .

Yesterday at sunset I was in a stony heath where some very small and twisted oaks grow, in the background a ruin on the hill and corn in the valley. It was romantic, like a Monticelli; the sun was pouring bright yellow rays upon the bushes and the ground, a perfect shower of gold, and all the lines were lovely.

And finally:

Now there is a glorious fierce heat, a sun, a light which for want of a better word I can only call yellow, pale sulphur yellow, pale lemon gold. How beautiful yellow is.

Life is almost an enchantment. Those who do not believe in the sun here are without faith!

To sum up, creativity appears to be more common among people with mood disorders, especially those whose condition is relatively mild, as well as among the relatives of such individuals. It is quite possible that genes for creativity and mood disorders are transmitted together. It is important for professionals who treat people with mood disorders to recognize this. Eradicating all mood swings may diminish creativity in some people, though it is likely to improve matters greatly for those whose mood swings are severe. Nowadays, when an understanding of the human genetic makeup is close at hand, and the possibility of preventing certain undesirable genes in new generations is scientifically conceivable, we would do well to consider the beneficial aspects of certain types of emotional disturbance, while never forgetting the pain they can cause.

SEVENTEEN

Winter Light

LIFE BEYOND SAD

One must have a mind for winter
To regard the frost and the boughs
Of the pine-trees crusted with snow;
And have been cold a long time
To behold the junipers shagged with ice,
The spruces rough in the distant glitter
Of the January sun; and not to think
Of any misery in the sound of the wind,
In the sound of a few leaves,
Which is the sound of the land
Full of the same wind
That is blowing in the same bare place
For the listener, who listens in the snow,
And, nothing himself, beholds
nothing that is not there and the nothing that is.
　　　　　—WALLACE STEVENS, "The Snow Man"

▶ Do you have a mind for winter, as this beautiful poem suggests?

▶ Are you ready to consider living life to the fullest during winter?

The joys of the season are not easily acquired, especially for those whose biology makes them want to flee from winter.

They are joys that must be earned. And so, gentle reader, having reached the end of this book, you have earned the right not only to endure winter, but to enjoy it; not only to treat the maladies that it brings, but to seek out its hidden pleasures. By now, we have a generation of people who have grown up since SAD was described and light therapy has been available. There are SAD veterans of many winters, those who have been unable or unwilling to flee to the sunny South but who have nevertheless made good lives for themselves in the North. I count myself among these fortunate individuals. This chapter deals with what we have learned about life beyond SAD and how we have found light in this dark season.

Winning My Own Battle with Winter

Winter no longer fills me with foreboding. All the evidence of its impending presence is still there in the world around me: the encroachment of dark at either end of the day, like a rat nibbling away at a piece of cheese; the leaves turning color; the odd angle of the sun. But the feeling is different. There is a stirring inside me, a sense that this is what I have been waiting for, the winter, a wild frontier, alien and familiar as the wilderness, provoking me to react, create, survive, and triumph. Perhaps that is what it feels like to raft down the white waters of an untamed river or scale a sheer cliff. I have no idea. I have never done either of these things and probably never will. No matter. Winter is adventure enough for me.

I have been told by rock climbers of the surge of adrenaline they feel when they gaze down hundreds of feet, especially those who hang from the cliff by their bare hands without the help of tools. I know of some who have even felt the need for such death-defying exploits to feel alive, a vital part of their world. Perhaps winter has offered that sort of adrenaline rush to humans ever since they wandered from the sun-drenched savannahs and ventured into the glacial regions of the North.

I was amazed to read of the ice man excavated from a glacier in which he had been buried for over 5,000 years. He was well equipped for life in that unfriendly climate. Dressed in bearskin clothes and a grass cape, he carried a copper ax and a bow and arrows, housed in a deerskin quiver. Among the many things found with the frozen man were two birch-bark canisters, which might have held the embers from a fire, a sloe berry—no doubt his food—and two mushrooms strung on a leather cord, perhaps a type of primitive antibiotic. Of course, no one is fully protected against bad luck, and all his tools and preparations were of no help to him on the fateful day of his death. I like to think that it was swift, a sudden blast of ice or snow and quick oblivion while he was asleep, dreaming of how best to snare some animal or find his favorite berries higher up the slopes. In any event, we are the beneficiaries of his untimely fate as nature, acting as museum curator, embalmed him for our scrutiny.

Harsh environments foster creativity, and winter in the North is about as harsh an environment as you can find on our planet. Animals that live at some distance from the equator must generate energy for all their body functions against the gradient of the freezing cold, when all the usual sources of energy in our physical world—plant and animal life—are at their lowest ebb. This challenge of survival is dramatized in the book *Two Old Women*, a moving story by Velma Wallis, in which she describes how two elders are abandoned by their tribe at the approach of winter. For these two frail people, being forced to confront the Alaskan winter without food, shelter, or electricity is virtually a death sentence. After absorbing the shock of this betrayal, one woman says, "If we are going to die, let us die trying, not sitting." And slowly, painfully, they try, compensating for their lack of strength and agility with a lifetime of accumulated wisdom and experience. Ultimately they succeed not only in surviving the winter but also in accumulating enough food to help feed the entire tribe.

Many people with SAD will surely be able to relate to the old women in Wallis's book. Even though you may not be old or live above the Arctic Circle,

Harsh environments foster creativity: Can you find a way to take advantage of the harshness of winter?

and though you may have adequate heat and food all year round, winter remains a difficult season. But as with the old women, the urge to fight against winter can triumph over the longing to give up and succumb to it. Nowadays, when asked how severe my SAD is, I am always at a loss for an answer, simply because for many years I have not allowed the condition its full expression. I have used every means at my disposal to overcome it, and as a consequence, each winter has become a little easier for me. Age and experience have been my allies, as have the examples of others who claim winter is the best time of year for them. I have tried to learn what they enjoy about winter so that I can experience it too. So far have my skills at managing the winter developed that I have even come to the point of looking forward to the winter, a state of mind I never thought possible.

One aspect of the winter that has been a source of joy for me is my research. Winter has been a critical part of my business. In this regard, I have found myself sharing an unexpected kinship with purveyors of space heaters, sweaters, and furs, with ice fishermen and ski instructors. I have researched the effects of darkness, and the success of such research depends on bad weather, which brings patients into a research program. Unseasonably clement winter weather, on the other hand, may keep potential research subjects away and may threaten studies by altering the biology of those involved in experiments. During one winter, my group did exceptionally well in recruiting patients for our program as the northeastern United States was hit by one ice storm after another. I would wake up each day, check the weather conditions, and respond with glee at the news of the latest storm. My wife was not amused.

Don't get me wrong, though. Such euphoria is not to be depended on, and winter still has the power to buffalo me. Every winter brings with it at least a few dark days when I feel a sort of stasis of the blood, a sludging of all my biological processes, especially my thinking. I am in slow motion in relation to the rest of the world and compared to how I feel at all other times of the year. I have come to accept these days, but I still dislike them. I wake up on such dark days stirring like a hedgehog disturbed from his hibernating state. I am in conservation mode and do and say only what is essential. Fortunately, with good self-care these days become fewer with each passing winter.

But when the winter stasis is upon me, I lose the capacity to process multiple things at the same time. I become linear. One idea has to be completed before there is room in my brain for the next one: One action at a time. Finish this before starting that. What a pain in the neck! So I proceed through my daily activities. Exercise is essential, coupled with light; yet motivation is hard to muster. On days of ice and snow, I work out on my elliptical trainer in front of a light box and some old favorite DVD.

By now, I have been through this cycle dozens of times since my arrival in North America. I understand its biological basis and, more important, that it will pass in time, provided I use light and exercise and limit the stresses that can be controlled. Above all, I need to accept my need to hibernate (albeit to a much reduced extent). I must let go of some of my driving demands. If I lower my expectations of myself, I have to acknowledge that my functioning is quite acceptable, and for now, that has to be good enough.

The holiday season brings its round of social activities. When I am not in my dark days, I am a very sociable person, but when the stasis of the blood sets in, I want to sit at home, to brood and ruminate. Now it is time for some dinner engagement, and I am paralyzed before my clothes closet, fixated over what shirt to pick out, over the ordinary things that have to be done to get out of the house and on my way. "I have no energy," I mutter under my breath. "I don't think I can possibly have any fun tonight."

But I usually do. People energize me. And so I am off again, carried forward by the remedies I both prescribe and use. And I do enjoy the parties, the friends, the fact that even though the sun has abandoned us yet again, there is still life to be had in winter. Or else, of an evening, I curl up with some good book, poetry perhaps, that can be read in snatches. On one occasion, my wife and I chose to spend New Year's Eve in the bedroom in front of the television. We had the bright lights on and dozed and watched television intermittently. And then, all of a sudden, "Auld Lang Syne" was playing and the ball was falling in Times Square. We gave each other a hug, and at that moment I had the distinct impression that somewhere in the heavens, the sun had passed its nadir and begun to climb.

Recapturing the Winters of Childhood

For most people who develop SAD, its symptoms begin after adolescence. Many of them have happy memories of the winters of their childhood, but these are buried under years of suffering. After they overcome their SAD symptoms, one of the unexpected gifts of this healing is to be able to access these memories once again and feel a sense of reintegration with their childhood selves. I have interviewed several such people with SAD who grew up in different parts of the United States, and here are three of their stories.

> SAD does not have to erase the joyful memories of your childhood winters. Addressing seasonality, in fact, allows you to reclaim that joy.

Skating in New England

The winters of New England, made famous in writings such as those of Robert Frost, are known for their snowy landscapes, icy paths, frigid temperatures, and the tough-mindedness of those who have made the region their home. Kathleen, now in her 30s, remembers growing up in Boston. For her, the joyful memories of winter are inextricably entangled with skating. She recalls:

> When I was 11 or so, I got my first pair of skates. There was a field nearby—technically more of a swamp—and in the fall, the boys would go down and burn up the field, and the fire department would come and put out the fire. All the reeds would have been burned down below the water level, and it would freeze over in the winter. We'd all go shovel it off and skate. The boys would play hockey, and the girls would try to do figure skating.
>
> We would occasionally get ice storms and ice would freeze on the trees, and it would be very dangerous. But one of the most fun memories I have of winter was of one such ice storm. Of course we didn't have school that day and the streets froze over to such an extent that we all grabbed our skates and went skating up and down the streets of the neighborhood and had a grand time.

As an adult, Kathleen controls her SAD well with a combination of light therapy and outdoor exercise. She continues to run, ski, and, of course, to skate. She notes:

> With skating, there comes a moment, after your body has warmed up and you're not rusty anymore, particularly if you are skating outdoors

and there are not a lot of people around, when everything comes together. I'm just skating, and there's the sky and the sun and the trees, and it's not even like praying anymore. I become the prayer. You become graceful, moving, but part of all the scene around you, the frozen pond, the soul of the trees and the sun.

Making a Wood Fire in Winter

Wood warms you twice—once when you cut it and once when it burns.
—HENRY DAVID THOREAU

James, a man in his 30s, formerly a mathematician, now owns and runs a flower and herb farm with his wife in the mid-Atlantic region of the United States. He recalls a lifelong love of wood fires in the winter.

We'd always have a fire when we got back home: that's always been a big thing for me. I love the fire in the fireplace. I like gathering and cutting the wood. It's almost as much fun as the fire itself. I've always liked the wood—the smell, the feel, cutting, organizing and stacking it, making use out of something that's already there, the resourcefulness of it. Not just turning on some kind of appliance. I like starting the fire in the fireplace, the challenge, knowing how to do it. You learn about bark, which wood not to burn, how to watch out for poison ivy, which you can get even worse in the winter than in the summer. I like cooking over fires and the direct heat of the fire, better than devices like heat pumps. I like its different phases or stages—as the thing dies down a little, it just sort of glows. A lot of times you'll get sleepy after a while; the fire kind of corresponds to your level of activity.

As an adult, James has handled his own seasonality by choosing a career that allows for varying levels of work at different times of year. He works with the sun—long hours in the summer and short hours in the winter. He has resisted growing too much in a greenhouse because that would defeat his wish to slow down during the winter. And there is no preserving, because everything fresh is purchased rapidly. He feels the changing seasons almost as he imagines a plant might feel them, waiting for the wild blackberries to come back each year and for the appearance of every fruit and flower at its predicted time. By fitting his lifestyle to his seasonal rhythms, James has found peace and contentment.

Drinking Tea in the Snow in Alaska

Beth, an Athapaskan Indian, was born in Alaska in a small village at the junction of the Yukon and Tanana Rivers. She recalls the special respect her people had for the land and all its animals, even those they hunted for sustenance. For example, when her brothers set out to kill a moose, they would never say out loud what they were planning to do. If they did, they believed, the moose would hear that boastful statement and evade them. Instead, they would say, "We're going to look around," and everyone knew what they meant. In the same way, telling a story about how they shot the moose would be frowned on.

Dealing with winter is a dominant theme in the lives of the Athapaskan Indians. The people would make intense preparations for the onset of winter. Beth's family would boat up to Fish Lake to pick the high- and lowbush cranberries to make jellies and jams for the winter. In late summer, they would catch salmon in fishnets and fish wheels and haul the salmon to the smokehouse so that it would last through the long winter months. Each family would shoot one moose at the start of the season. You shot only as much as you needed—no more.

Winters were tough in many ways. The family had only a wood-stove for warmth and cooking. Beth's father and brothers would go out to cut birchwood, often in the waist-deep snow, wearing caribou-skin boots tied with leather thongs below the knees. For additional food, they would hunt ptarmigan and rabbit in the snow.

Beth and her friends enjoyed outdoor things, even though at mid-winter in Alaska there were only 4 hours of light a day. The lake would freeze over, smooth as a mirror, and they would skate on it or go sledding. They would hitch up the dogs and sled into the woods to build a campfire, make tea, and drink it with crackers and dry fish. Those were peaceful times.

Night was a time for visiting, telling funny stories, and playing wild card games in which the cards flew about in all directions. Then there were special occasions, when family-oriented activities and square dances would take place. She remembers winters as a time enjoyed by all.

Nothing in her childhood would have prepared Beth for the onset, later in life, of seasonal depression, inherited perhaps from her Caucasian father, who had married an Athapaskan woman. For this she was treated successfully with light therapy. She moved to Colorado, which she thought would be better for her because of the greater abundance of light at that lower latitude. Feeling culturally isolated from her people, however, she elected to return to Alaska, where she currently works and functions well throughout the year. Back in Anchorage, she is close to her family, her traditions, and her personal history, which she can now enjoy all winter long thanks to brief post-Christmas vacations in Mexico and the successful treatment of her SAD symptoms.

The Joys of Winter

As the preceding stories indicate, many joys can be found in winter, if only one has the inclination and energy to seek them. Here are some that I have encountered during winters in the North. I encourage you to pursue all forms of healthy pleasure in the dark season.

Festivals, Stories, and Gifts

Winter is a fine time for festivals, storytelling, and gifts. Given the natural dreariness of the season, it is not surprising that different cultures have chosen to celebrate this time of year with festivals, many of which have ancient origins. Christmas, for example, is said to have its roots in pagan times, Hanukkah to hark back to the time of the Maccabees. Aside from these winter solstice festivals, there are a host of other ritualized celebrations to cheer up the dark days: Halloween, Thanksgiving, Oktoberfest, Valentine's Day, Groundhog Day, and the Ice Festival are all ways of marking the passing of winter in a spirited manner. According to one Minnesotan I spoke with, "The Ice Festival is a time when we go out and shake our fists at winter."

Giving and receiving gifts is a great way of remembering that we love and are loved even during winter. They are a natural addition to the winter festivals. Sometimes the best gifts are those that cost very little but mean a great deal. For example, one winter holiday when an ice storm caused our pipes to burst, I called a friend who is a building contractor, lamenting this sorry turn of events. He came right over, and we set out together to the hardware store to purchase the parts needed to fix the pipes. My friend, who would much rather be a teacher than a contractor, decided it was a good opportunity to beef up my home-improvement skills. He guided me through the steps involved in fixing the pipes and, to my amazement, I did it! Afterwards, we celebrated this accomplishment together over a Chinese dinner.

Another time, over a Christmas lunch with my friend Kay Redfield Jamison, we traded our usual gifts. The one I remember most, though, from that day was the story she told me of the characters Rat and Mole from Kenneth Grahame's *The Wind in the Willows*—a story of friendship between two small creatures caught in a snowstorm. After lunch, she insisted on taking me to the nearest bookstore to buy a copy of the book that related this tale of empathy and understanding between friends on a winter's day.

So stories can be gifts and gifts can generate stories, and both are excellent ways of bringing joy to the dark season. One of the most famous Christmas stories that connects giving with the season is O. Henry's "The Gift of the Magi," in which a husband and wife each sacrifice a prized possession to purchase a gift for the other. The husband sells his watch to buy combs for his wife's hair; she sells her hair to buy a chain for his watch. The story illustrates how love itself is a great gift, surpassing material possessions—a message that helps us look beyond the material and into the spiritual, a message consistent with the spirit of winter.

It is not only in Western culture that storytelling thrives in winter. Among the Lenape Indians, for example, the time for storytelling began with the first frost and ended with the last frost. The Indians were superstitious about telling stories during the summer for fear that the creatures of the forest might hear the storyteller talking about them and take revenge on him. Or the crops might stop and listen to the storyteller and forget to grow. They believed that stories carry great power—and so do we, as evidenced by how far people are willing to go out of their way for a well-told story on stage or screen. The most powerful stories are those that stay with us and continue to affect us long after the last word is spoken or the last sentence read.

In some cultures and climates, for example in the Far North, gifts in winter can make the difference between life and death. Beth, the

Athapaskan woman mentioned earlier, told me how in her village they always saw to it that no one went through the winter without enough food to eat. Psychiatrist Andrés Magnusson remembers how in the town in Iceland where he grew up they would round up the homeless on Christmas Eve and take them to the jail, where they would be sure to be warm and have a decent meal. Even farther south, we are enjoined around Christmastime to remember the neediest. There is something about this season of scarcity that brings out the best in us: witness the transformation of Ebenezer Scrooge in the perennial classic *A Christmas Carol*.

Other Pleasures

Once the symptoms of SAD have been treated, even if only partially, all kinds of winter pleasures become possible, such as sports, socializing, reading, travel, solitude, and walking.

For the sports fan, winter presents many opportunities for both observing and participating. It is basketball and Super Bowl season for those whose preferred position is on the couch in front of the television. For the more active, snow and ice offer many opportunities for physical exercise, and the glittering light reflected off snowy surfaces is sure to elevate the spirits further.

When the symptoms of SAD are treated, thinking becomes sharper and it is easier to read again, to concentrate on another person's thoughts. Curling up in front of the fireplace with a good book can be a special treat on a winter day. You can even read about winter itself. To the untreated SAD sufferer, such books may provide cold comfort, but once symptoms are treated, they may spark your interest. Edwin Way Teale, in his prize-winning *Traveling through Winter*, describes winter as "a hundred seasons in one." In his charming book *Winter*, Rick Bass chronicles how he traveled to Montana to experience winter in the North. We read how he rides out his SAD-like symptoms, which he regards as part of the authentic winter experience. Donald Hall, in an essay on winter, describes himself as a lover of winter, "partly tuber, partly bear."

Perhaps more poetry has been written about winter than about any other season. One good thing about poetry is that it's short and therefore doesn't unduly tax one's attention span, which may be a boon for someone suffering from SAD. Japanese haiku may be particularly appealing at this time, because each poem has only seventeen syllables. Somehow, in the spareness of the wording and references to nature, winter haiku has an amazing capacity to evoke the beauty, peace, and solitude of the season. Although winter is a season of parties and socializing, it is also conducive to solitude, whether for the reader by the fire or the skier on the slopes. In this regard as well, it is a season of contrasts.

Although stressful travel should be avoided during winter if you have SAD, once your symptoms are relatively well controlled, travel in winter can also be a great diversion. I am not referring only to escaping winter by heading south, but also to traveling through and sometimes even into winter. One such trip that I took was a book tour to some of the darkest cities in the United States. With the help of the light visor, I not only was able to get through the trip successfully but actually managed to enjoy it as well.

Winter can surprise. For example, when I reached Seattle, one of the darkest cities in the country, this beautiful town was awash in dazzling sunshine. There were clear views of the Cascade and Olympic mountain ranges, and not a cloud was to be seen over the huge Mount Rainier. As I think of that day, I can still see the turquoise color of the sky that to me typifies the mystical beauty of the Pacific Northwest.

In Portland, Oregon, on the other hand, where it rarely snows, I arrived in the midst of the first snowstorm in a very long time. The flakes were small and feathery at first but later turned into a blizzard that paralyzed a city ill equipped to deal with it. Luckily, my tour guide had a four-wheel-drive SUV, so I was able to enjoy the way the snow had transformed the landscape, frosting the gingerbread roofs of the Victorian houses and freighting down the blackberry canes with cotton-white mounds. The sculpted fir trees, tufted with snow, were still festooned with red tinsel streamers from the holiday season. Red, white, and green: the official colors of Christmas. From the city park, a bronze deer, icicles hanging from its nose, gazed out at me, unmoved by the wintry spectacle.

The day of interviews went off without a hitch despite the weather, thanks to both my intrepid guide and the tenacity of the journalists involved, all of whom had gamely made it to their stations. By the day's end, the snow had turned to slush, and as I stepped into the truck I could see the brilliant reds and golds of autumn leaves shining through the melting crystals. The words of Albert Camus came to mind: "Even in the midst of winter, there is within me an invincible summer."

> *This is the challenge of winter: somehow to hold on to our reserves of hope, cheer, and energy even when the dark and the cold drain us of much of our good humor and vitality.*

Thoreau has written about the special joy of walking in winter. It is a joy I share with him. Although life may seem to have largely deserted the cities, there is much to be seen in the wilderness and parklands all around. The architecture of the trees can be appreciated best without their summer greenery. Where flowers once bloomed, the winter weeds hold on to their intricately crafted seed cases. Many birds remain behind in the North. In Maryland, for example, there are chickadees, Canada geese (not all of which migrate to the far South), great blue herons, scarlet cardinals, and bald eagles. Pairs of eagles will return to build their nest in the same location, year after year, in January and have their young in February. You can hear the sound of water running over stones, fed by underground streams or ice cracking at the edge of a pond. Deer and foxes roam between rocks covered with moss and lichen, as green as jade.

You may not need to stray far to enjoy walking in winter. As I walk through the familiar streets of my own neighborhood, I am reminded of how the different gardens looked last summer and compare that with their present dormancy. I enjoy the purple hearts of decorative cabbages or the red berries of holly at a time of year when any flash of color provides a welcome relief against the background of grays, browns, and conifer green. The air has a bracing quality.

Winter nights are especially good for walking and for stargazing when it is cloudless. One winter night, I stared through a telescope and saw the moons of Jupiter and the rings of Saturn for the first time. And often, when the chill is not too forbidding, as I wander through the quiet suburban streets, I think of "Winter Heavens," a poem by George Meredith:

Sharp is the night, but stars with frost alive
Leap off the rim of earth across the dome
It is a night to make the heavens our home

More than the nest whereto apace we strive.
Lengths down our road each fir-tree seems a hive,
In swarms outrushing from the golden comb.
They waken waves of thoughts that burst to foam.

The darkness of the night is broken by the stars and the light of human habitation—streetlights, incandescent lights, flickering television screens, computer terminals, and, at the end of my walk, the bright cheerful lights shining through the curtains of my own home. And as I return to the beginning again, I think of winter and its many, many facets. It has been a difficult season, for me and so very many others, but in the difficulty there is the opportunity to bring out that which is best in each of us. Winter is a stimulus to creativity and to sharing the fruits of our creation with others. I write this book in that spirit, and if it brings you even a shaft of light on a winter's day, my mission has been accomplished.

Part IV

Resources

WEBSITES OF INTEREST

www.normanrosenthal.com
My personal website. I provide regular blogs and updates on SAD and its treatment, as well as other aspects of my work.

www.cet.org
An excellent all-around Web resource is run by the Center for Environmental Therapeutics.

www.chronotherapeutics.org/forum_eng.html
The listserv of *cet.org.*

www.pubmed.org
For scholars, I recommend the website for the National Library of Medicine, an invaluable resource. Just punch in one or more subjects or authors of interest and the relevant articles will appear. Usually, you will get the abstract of the article free. If you need the full article, either you need to have access to a university or other organization with that privilege or you can set up an account and pay for the articles. Having this kind of resource at your disposal has made it unnecessary for me to list many of the articles mentioned in the book, which can be accessed using the name of the lead authors. Those who are interested might want to check out the original articles.

www.sltbr.org
The website for the Society for Light Therapy and Biological Rhythms. Includes information in the Society's annual meeting.

www.beckinstitute.org
The website for the Beck Institute for Cognitive Behavior Therapy.

www.academyofct.org
The website for the Academy of Cognitive Therapy.

www.tm.org
www.davidlynchfoundation.org
Information on transcendental meditation.

www.mindfulselfcompassion.org
Christopher Germer's website. Includes downloads of mindfulness exercises.

WHERE TO OBTAIN LIGHT FIXTURES AND OTHER DEVICES

In Chapter 7 I have provided general guidelines for choosing a suitable light box or dawn simulator. I recommend that you read them before making your choice. The pictures in the chapter show some of the fixtures I have found helpful and appealing, along with their manufacturers. These manufacturers have a long track record for quality control, reliability, and willingness to stand by their products. Contact information for them is listed below. There are, however, other good companies with products on the market, and you may well prefer a different type of fixture or another manufacturer; you should be able to obtain the fixture you prefer via the Internet. In all instances, make sure the company offers a full money-back guarantee within 30 days if you are not satisfied with the product for any reason.

Verilux, Inc.
Healthy Lighting Company
340 Mad River Park
Waitsfield, VT 05673
Phone: 802-496-3101
Toll-free: 800-454-4408
Fax: 802-496-3105
www.verilux.com

SunBox Company
19217 Orbit Drive
Gaithersburg, MD 20879
Phone: 301-869-5980
Toll-free: 800-LITE-YOU (548-3968)
www.sunbox.com
E-mail: info@sunbox.com
   Besides light boxes, dawn simulators, light visors, and light pipes, negative ion generators can also be obtained from SunBox.

BioBrite, Inc.
4330 East-West Highway
Suite 310
Bethesda, MD 20814
Toll-free: 800-621-LITE
www.biobrite.com
E-mail: support@biobrite.com

SUPPORT GROUPS

Support Groups for SAD

The longest-standing support group for seasonal affective disorder is the SAD Association of Great Britain (SADA), which has been in operation for decades, during which it has served hundreds of thousands of people. It is an exemplary nonprofit organization that is well worth looking into, especially if you live in the United Kingdom. Its contact information is shown below.

Seasonal Affective Disorder Association (SADA)
P.O. Box 989
Steyning BN44 3HG, United Kingdom
www.sada.org.uk

In many instances a support group can be established through the persistence of a single individual, who then inspires many others to follow her or his example. In the case of SADA, Jennifer Eastwood was the founding member, though dozens of dedicated volunteers have kept the organization going since its inception.

More recently, Esther O'Hara, formerly of the United Kingdom and now living in Sweden, appealed to SADA to help her start a Swedish support group. Contact information for Esther and her group are shown below.

SAD in Sweden
www.sadinsweden.com
Esther O'Hara
Von Döbelns Väg 56
Trollhättan 461 58, Sweden
E-mail: estherohara@gmail.com

Support Groups for Mood Disorders and Other Emotional Disorders

Depression and Bipolar Support Alliance (DBSA; formerly known as National Depressive and Manic–Depressive Association [NMDA])
730 North Franklin Street, Suite 501
Chicago, IL 60610-7224
Toll-free: 800-826-3632
www.dbsalliance.org

National Alliance on Mentally Illness (NAMI)
Colonial Place Three
2107 Wilson Boulevard, Suite 300
Arlington, VA 22201-3042
Phone: 703-524-7600 (main)
Toll-free: 888-999-6264 (member services)
www.nami.org

FURTHER READING

General Readings on SAD, Light Therapy, and Related Topics

Lam, R. W. (1998). *Seasonal affective disorder and beyond: Light treatment for SAD and non-SAD conditions.* Washington, DC: American Psychiatric Press.

Lam, R. W., & Levitt, A. J. (Eds.). (1999). *Clinical guidelines for the treatment of seasonal affective disorder.* Vancouver: Clinical and Academic Publishing.

Oren, D. A., Reich, W., Rosenthal, N. E., & Wehr, T. A. (2006). *How to beat jet lag: A practical guide for air travelers.* New York: Henry Holt.

Partonen, T., & Pandi-Perumm S. R. (Eds.). (2010). *Seasonal affective disorder: Practice and research* (2nd ed.). New York: Oxford University Press.—A comprehensive but technical book; will be of value mainly to scholars.

Rosenthal, N. E., & Blehar, M. C. (Eds.). (1989). *Seasonal affective disorders and phototherapy.* New York: Guilford Press.—The first compilation of papers on SAD and light therapy, including chapters on the history of SAD and other aspects of the early thinking on the subject; will be of interest to scholars.

Rosenthal, N. E., Sack, D. A., Gillin, J. C., Lewy, A. J., Goodwin, F. K., Davenport, Y., et al. (1984). Seasonal affective disorder: A description of the syndrome and preliminary findings with light therapy. *Archives of General Psychiatry, 41*(1), 72–80.—The original description of SAD and its treatment with light therapy.

Terman, M., & McMahan, I. (2012). *Chronotherapy: Resetting your inner clock to boost mood, alertness, and quality sleep.* New York, Avery/Penguin.

Wehr, T. A., et al. (2001). A circadian signal of change of season in patients with seasonal affective disorder. *Archives of General Psychiatry, 58*(12), 1108–1114.

Wirz-Justice, A., Benedetti, F., & Terman, M. (2009). *Chronotherapeutics for affective disorders: A clinician's manual for light and wake therapy.* Basel, Switzerland: Karger.

Diet and SAD

Bowden, J. (2005). *Living low-carb: Controlled carbohydrate eating for long-term weight loss.* New York: Sterling.

Peeke, P. (2012). *The hunger fix: The three-stage detox and recovery plan for overeating and food addiction.* Emmans, PA: Rodale.

Willett, W. C. (2005). *Eat, drink and be healthy: The Harvard Medical School guide to healthy eating.* New York: Free Press.

Psychotherapy for SAD

Rohan, K. J. (2008). *Coping with the seasons: A cognitive-behavioral approach to seasonal affective disorder (Workbook).* New York: Oxford University Press.

Meditation for SAD

Ekirch, A. R. (2005). *At day's close: Night in times past.* New York: Norton.

Germer, C. K. (2009). *The mindful path to self-compassion: Freeing yourself from destructive thoughts and emotions.* New York: Guilford Press.

Gunaratana, B. H. (2011). *Mindfulness in plain English* (20th anniv. ed.). Somerville, MA: Wisdom Publications.

Hofman, S. G., Sawyer, A. T., Witt, A. A., & Ph, D. (2010). The effect of mindfulness-based therapy on anxiety and depression: A meta-analytic review. *Journal of Consulting and Clinical Psychology, 78*(2), 169–183.

Rosenthal, N. E. (2011). *Transcendence: Healing and transformation through transcendental meditation.* New York: Tarcher Penguin.

Shear, J. (Ed.). (2006). *The experience of meditation: Experts introduce the major traditions.* St. Paul, MN: Paragon House.

Siegel, R. D. (2010). *The mindfulness solution: Everyday practices for everyday problems.* New York: Guilford Press.

Warren, J. (2007). *The head trip: Adventures on the wheel of consciousness.* New York: Random House.

Williams, M., Teasdale, J., Segal, Z., & Kabat-Zinn, J. (2007). *The mindful way through depression: Freeing yourself from chronic unhappiness.* New York: Guilford Press.

APPENDIX A

Daily Mood Log

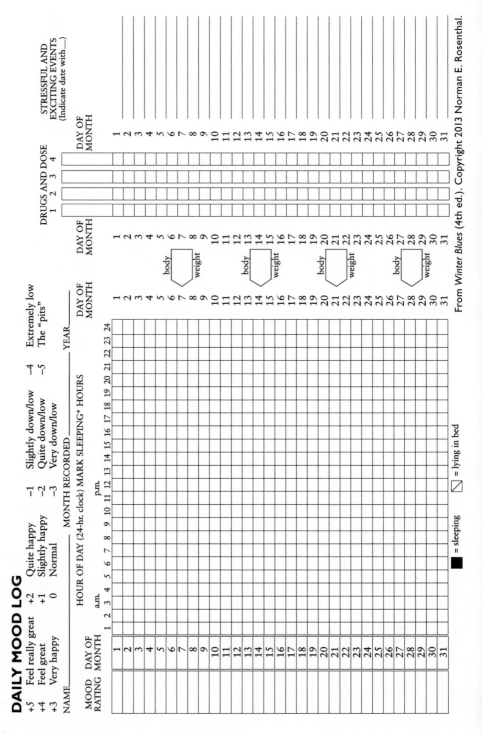

From *Winter Blues* (4th ed.). Copyright 2013 Norman E. Rosenthal.

328

Core Belief Worksheet

CORE BELIEF WORKSHEET

Name: _____ Date: _____

Old core belief: _____

_____

- How much do you believe the old core belief right now? (0–100)___
- What's the most you've believed it this week? (0–100)___
- What's the least you've believed it this week? (0–100)___

New belief: _____

_____

- How much do you believe the new belief right now? (0–100)___

Evidence that contradicts old core belief and supports new belief	Evidence that seems to support old core belief with reframe

Should situations related to an increase or decrease in the strength of the belief be topics for the agenda?

Acknowledgments

Space doesn't permit me to acknowledge all those who helped make this book possible. Many contributed their stories anonymously and therefore must be thanked off the record. Special thanks, however, are due to Thomas Wehr, David Sack, Dan Oren, Fred Jacobsen, Paul Schwartz, Leo Sher, and Erick Turner, my principal colleagues at the National Institute of Mental Health, for our many creative interactions that helped shape my thinking. Other colleagues who have been exceptionally generous in sharing their thoughts and research findings are Michael and Jiuan-Su Terman, Siegfried Kasper, Raymond Lam, Alfred Lewy, Kelly Rohan, George Brainard, Charmane Eastman, Barbara Parry, Jack Modell, and Elizabeth Wehr. For their help in advancing my understanding of meditation, I wish to thank Robert Roth, Fred Travis, Robert Schneider, Mario Orsatti, Linda Mainquist, David Orme-Johnson, Chris Germer, and Zindel Segal. Thanks to my editors at The Guilford Press, Seymour Weingarten, Kitty Moore, and Chris Benton, who have been uniformly outstanding and supportive. Thanks also to my personal editor and friend Elise Hancock. The light box companies whose products are shown in Chapter 7 were unfailingly helpful. I am grateful to all my colleagues in the field of SAD and light therapy, who have provided inspiration and fellowship over the past decades. Many are mentioned in this book. Finally, I owe a huge debt to Leora and Josh for their support over the years.

The following publishers have generously given permission to use extended quotations from copyrighted works:

From *Cognitive Therapy: Basics and Beyond* (p. 177), by Judith S. Beck. Copyright 1993 by Judith S. Beck. Reprinted by permission of The Guilford Press.

From *Diagnostic and Statistical Manual of Mental Disorders* (4th edition, text revision), by the American Psychiatric Association. Copyright 2000 by the American Psychiatric Association. Reprinted by permission.

From *Japanese Haiku: Two Hundred Twenty Examples of Seventeen-Syllable Poems* (p. 60), translated by Peter Bellenson. Copyright 2008 by Bibliobazaar. Reprinted by permission of Peter Pauper Press, Inc.

From *The Letters of Henry Adams, Volume II* (pp. 51–52), edited by J. C. Levenson, Ernest Samuels, Charles Vendersee, and Viola Hopkins Winner. Copyright 1982 by the Massachusetts Historical Society. Reprinted by permission of the Belknap Press of Harvard University Press.

From *Selected Letters of Gustav Mahler*, by Gustav Mahler. Copyright 1979 by Gustav Mahler. Reprinted by permission of Farrar, Straus and Giroux, LLC, and Faber and Faber Ltd.

From "The Snow Man" in *The Collected Poems of Wallace Stevens*, by Wallace Stevens. Copyright 1954 by Wallace Stevens and renewed 1982 by Holly Stevens. Reprinted by permission of Alfred A. Knopf, a division of Random House, Inc.; Faber and Faber Ltd.; and Pollinger Ltd.

The photographs in Figures 3 through 8 were generously provided by and used by permission of the SunBox Company, Gaithersburg, Maryland; Verilux, Inc., St. Paul, Minnesota; Northern Light Technologies, Montreal, Quebec, Canada; and the Center for Environmental Therapeutics, Zug, Switzerland.

Index

Parry, Barbara, 168, 331
Paxil (paroxetine), 219*t*, 225. *See also*
    Antidepressants
Personalization type of cognitive
    distortion, 206
Pessimism, 192
Pets, 148
Phase response curve, 164
Photopigments, 137–138
Physical complaints, 90
Physical environment, effect of,
    114–115, 130, 305
Physical illness, 235–236. *See* Illness
Playwrights, mental illness among,
    295
Pleasant activities
    annual cycle of symptoms and, 273
    CBT and, 201
Pleasure, 224, 273
Pleeter, J., 87*f*
PMDD (premenstrual dysphoric
    disorder). *See* Premenstrual
    difficulties
PMS. *See* Premenstrual difficulties
Poetry, 294, 298, 307, 313
Positive ions, 188–189. *See also*
    Negative ions
Postolache, Teodor, 61, 138–139
Practice
    CBT and, 197–199
    challenging your core negative
    beliefs, 209–210
Pregnancy, 147
Premenstrual difficulties
    examples of, 168–170
    light therapy and, 168–170
    overview, 43–44
Productivity, seasonality and, 295
Professional help. *See also*
    Cognitive-behavioral therapy;
    Psychotherapy; Treatment

choosing a psychotherapist,
    211–213
light therapy and, 121, 124
overview, 3–4
when to consider, 59–61, 195–196
Progesterone, 68
Prolactin, 74, 234
Prozac (fluoxetine), 80, 91, 103,
    104, 160, 219*t*, 225. *See also*
    Antidepressants
Psychiatric disorders
    light therapy and, 167–170
    link of with creativity, 294–297
    support groups for, 323
Psychotherapy. *See also* Cognitive-
    behavioral therapy; Professional
    help; Treatment
    choosing a psychotherapist,
    211–213
    further reading, 325
    overview, 194, 210–211
    when to consider, 195–196
Ptarmigan, 74, 310
Puberty, 63, 86
Putilov, Arcady, 176

Q

Questions in CBT, 207–208

R

Racing thoughts, 109, 141
Rape, 112
The Reaper, 300
Reddening of the skin, 142. *See also*
    Skin health
Reindeer, seasonal rhythms in,
    74–75
Relapse
    CBT and, 210

About the Author

Norman E. Rosenthal, MD, is internationally recognized for his pioneering contributions to understanding SAD and using light therapy to treat it. He is Clinical Professor of Psychiatry at Georgetown Medical School, a therapist in private practice, and the author of five books, including *Transcendence: Healing and Transformation through Transcendental Meditation.* Dr. Rosenthal conducted research at the National Institute of Mental Health for over 20 years.